AFTER *the* CRASH

HOW TO KEEP YOUR JOB, STAY IN SCHOOL, AND LIVE LIFE AFTER A BRAIN INJURY

KELLY TUTTLE FNP-BC, MSN

NEUROLOGY NURSE PRACTITIONER

Copyright © 2022 Kelly Tuttle

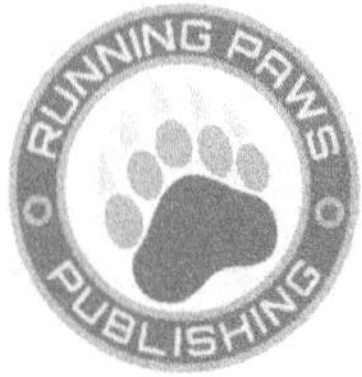

Running Paws Publishing
kellytuttlenp@gmail.com

ISBN: 979-8-9865095-0-1 (paperback)
ISBN: 979-8-9865095-1-8 (ebook)
ISBN: 979-8-9865095-2-5 (hardcover)
ISBN: 979-8-9865095-3-2 (audiobook)

Ordering Information:
Special discounts are available on quantity purchases by corporations, associations, and others. For details, contact kellytuttlenp@gmail.com

Table of Contents

SECTION I: INTRODUCTION

Chapter 1   Living with a Stranger 3

SECTION II: SYMPTOMS

Chapter 2   Common Symptoms after a Head Injury 15

Chapter 3   Vision A Not-So-Fun Fun House 21

Chapter 4   Hearing It's a Loud, Loud, Loud, Loud World 29

Chapter 5   Communication Breakdown Star Trek versus Starbucks 35

Chapter 6   Dizziness I'm Not Drunk! 41

Chapter 7   Headaches Living with Torture 49

Chapter 8   Fatigue A Constant, Cruel Companion 55

Chapter 9   Your Inner Hulk Behavior Changes after a Head Injury 63

SECTION III: TOOLS AND STRATEGIES

Chapter 10   My Tool Bag 73

Chapter 11   Journaling Yes, You're Making Progress:
It's Right There in Writing 75

Chapter 12   Tools for Work and School Light and Sound 81

Chapter 13   The Tornado Learning to Multitask with a Brain Injury 91

Chapter 14   Don't Break Your Brain—Give It a Brain Break 103

Chapter 15   Getting Off on the Wrong Foot
I'm Late, I'm Late, for a Very Important Date! 115

Chapter 16   Managing Your To-Do List: I'm Sorry. What Memory? 123

Chapter 17   Learning How to Learn Again 137

SECTION IV: LIFESTYLE

Chapter 18   Lifestyle Live Long and Prosper 145

Chapter 19   Sleep Is the Foundation of Recovery 147

Chapter 20   Mindfulness 153

Chapter 21   Exercise 161

Chapter 22   The Best Nutrition for Your Brain 167

Chapter 23   Protecting Your Livelihood and Finances 177

SECTION V: GETTING BACK TO LIFE

Chapter 24   Getting Back Behind the Wheel 189

This book is dedicated to those whose lives were changed in a moment, who feel lost in their own heads and are barely getting through each day. Remember, you are a badass. You survived what has killed others. And you are not alone.

Section I

Introduction

Chapter 1

Living with a Stranger

EVERY DAY, I LIVE with a stranger inside my head.

At first, I didn't know who she was. I just knew I didn't like her.

She was self-centered, emotionally immature, and easily distracted, and she slept all the time. She was annoyingly unmotivated and disorganized. She couldn't arrive on time to an appointment. She was a jerk who cussed too much, got angry easily, and dominated conversations. She couldn't remember anything and made it hard for me to think straight. On really bad days when I was exhausted and mentally spent, she would whisper to me that I was a stupid failure, reminding me that nothing I did would ever be good enough. She even made me believe that everyone would be better off if I just ended my life.

It took me three months to realize this stranger had hijacked my brain and was distorting my personality and perceptions. It was at this time that I started to reassert control over her. But even then, the stranger did not dissipate, and for a few years, I secretly lived with her feeding me thoughts. Often, I kept this hidden from my family and friends. At first her thoughts were the loud, prominent thoughts of my mind. Fortunately as time passed, these disturbing ideas and cognitions faded as my head injury healed.

Years later, I no longer consider her a stranger.

She is my new brain.

Before we go any further, I want to first say that I'm so sorry you find yourself reading this book if it means you've sustained a head injury and aren't better yet or if you know someone who is struggling to get better.

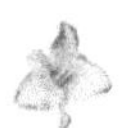

You are not alone. A Centers for Disease Control and Prevention (CDC) report to Congress in 2015 estimated between 3.2 and 5.3 million people in the U.S. live with disabilities caused by traumatic brain injuries.[1] So, hello and welcome to the head injury survivors club. Any time you share that you have had a head injury, you might be surprised at how many others have one too and how many others are affected by these people, including co-workers, friends, and loved ones.

I spent years trying to return to my former self without realizing I was never going to be that person again. I was an energetic, goal-driven individual who enjoyed spending time with my family and volunteering. I loved to snowboard, go to concerts, and travel with my husband and two daughters. One of my favorite things to do was hop in my car and spend hours exploring a new beach or town over a weekend. I relished making to-do lists and often created new goals, checking them off as I accomplished them. I would work all day and then fill my evenings practicing martial arts, having dinner with friends, or attending professional gatherings.

After my head injury, I watched all of my energy, passion, and drive just fly right out the window. Does this sound familiar?

---

[1] Centers for Disease Control and Prevention, *Traumatic Brain Injury in the United States: Epidemiology and Rehabilitation*, 2015, https://www.cdc.gov/traumaticbraininjury/pdf/TBI_Report_to_Congress_Epi_and_Rehab-a.pdf.

I often wondered, as many do, when I would get "better." I struggled with my short-term memory. I couldn't focus on anything. I drifted through days and didn't accomplish anything, which only worsened my frustration and anxiety.

I'm here to tell you that, after some wrecked relationships, poor decision-making, and months of wondering if I would get better, I crumpled up my life plans and hammered out a balance between my new passions and my residual capabilities. There is hope. I did get better, and you can too.

In this book, you'll find all the tools, strategies, and information that I used not necessarily to "heal" myself but to learn how to adapt. Throughout my process of recovery, I learned how to shape my life to my new brain. I developed tools and strategies that I could use to ensure I was staying on top of my professional and personal responsibilities and wasn't forgetting important deadlines.

In order to do this, I had to overhaul my entire life. I had to reorganize everything I did throughout my day. I had to change my exercise routine and even my sleep habits. I had to learn how to live with that total stranger in my head. The process took me nearly six years, but it worked. I learned to live with my head injury and deal with the stranger inside my head. Together, we became the new me.

The Car Accident

My story starts with the horrible sound of screeching rubber, followed by the unnatural, thunderous clap of metal. I felt as if Jet Li had simultaneously punched me in the face and kicked me in the chest. The latter were the airbags that saved my life.

Once the smoke cleared, I realized a teenage driver pulled out in front of me while I was driving down a rural road. It was June 23, 2015. At the time, I was 47 years old and the mother of two young daughters. The accident occurred in the evening as I was driving to karate class after leaving work as a cardiology nurse practitioner. Fortunately for both of us, we were in well-made German cars. Though we both survived, my cute little black Mercedes sports car was a smoky, smashed wreck.

In a daze, I declined being taken to the ER by ambulance, thinking that I was okay and would be able to shake this crash off in a few days. I was the type of person who had no patience for rest and who didn't know what it meant "to take it easy." I would, from that day forward, have to learn.

It wasn't until three months later that I realized something was seriously wrong with me. A friend of mine encouraged me to return to my third-degree black belt training. While there, I found that I struggled when I would try to perform a kata, a series of coordinated martial arts moves that I had performed numerous times in the past. Now I was struggling to even remember the moves. Normally, I would hear my instructor call out the name of a kata, and I would perform it quickly and smoothly, relying mostly on muscle memory. I was surprised to find myself standing there like a deer in the headlights, trying to remember the movements.

When I did remember the moves, I realized that even if I wanted my foot to move forward, my brain would make it step back. I would get frustrated and try to concentrate harder, but this seemed to make my memory freeze up and to make the communication between me and my body worse. To top it off, halfway through the kata, I noticed shortness of breath, and my arms and legs felt weak. I was used to working out for hours, and now I found myself with a pounding headache, neck pain, and exhaustion after only two minutes of training, causing me to become further frustrated.

When I could not return to my martial arts training and failed my third-degree black belt test, it finally clicked. Something was wrong with my brain. Something was wrong with me.

It was the first time I connected my struggles with concentration and fatigue with my head injury. Could this be due to my concussion? How could that be? In my mind, enough time had passed that I felt I should've been recovered from the incident. Later that day, I went home and reread the information I'd found on the internet about recovering from a head injury. I learned that the symptoms I was struggling with were all there, listed in the articles: fatigue, lack of concentration, headaches, and all the others. How could it be that three months after my car accident I was getting worse instead of better?

I was frantic to find information about how to recover from my concussion and was frustrated to find the answers I sought were elusive and not specific to my needs. You may have found, like me, information for military personnel, athletes, kids, teenagers, and other people who have suffered moderate to severe traumatic brain injuries. But where was the information for regular people like me?

Types of Head Injuries

After researching, I learned you can sustain a head injury in numerous ways: falling, having an object strike your head, crashing your car, playing sports, getting into a bar brawl, or being exposed to a blast while serving in the military. Head injuries can include bleeding in the brain (also called hemorrhages, which are small blood vessel leaks), a contusion (localized bruising of brain tissue), or the more general, widespread damage seen with most concussions.

Following a head injury, you may be told you have a mild head injury, concussion, or mild traumatic brain injury. These diagnoses are often interchangeable both by researchers and clinical professionals. If your head injury symptoms persist beyond a few weeks, you may be told that you have post-concussion syndrome.

Just keep in mind that there's no test that will definitively diagnose you with a mild traumatic brain injury (TBI) or concussion. Head CT scans and brain MRIs will show gross structural brain damage, a skull fracture, or bleeding in the brain. What these scans are not capable of demonstrating is damage to your brain at the cellular level, and this is the level where head injury symptoms originate.

Though getting a head CT or brain MRI can be reassuring, don't be surprised if it's normal. Even if your test results come back normal, you can still have suffered from a concussion or mild TBI. You also don't have to suffer a coma, loss of consciousness, or be hospitalized for a head injury for the TBI to have a significant impact on your life. Therefore, your symptoms are real, and it's important that you get the medical care you and your brain need.

At first, I was told by my general practitioner that I had a concussion. A couple months later, it was changed to post-concussion syndrome. Later, six months after the crash, I was told I had a TBI because the car accident slammed my brain back and forth between the front and the back of my skull, tearing the delicate connecting fibers between my brain cells. Throughout this book I will use the term head injury or brain injury to keep things simple.

RECOVERY TIMELINE

Prior to a head injury, most people probably never gave their brain a second thought. This is because you coexisted as one—the brain and the body working in harmony. But after a head injury, it can feel as if you've suddenly been severed from yourself, becoming a team of two: there's you, and then there's your brain. For me, it seemed as if my brain had taken over.

As you may have also noticed, there often seems to be something blocking your path to recovery that prevents you from returning to your old life. Well, you're correct, as it's common for your brain to pull on the reins. It's your brain's way of saying, "No, we need to rest, heal, and figure out how to go forward."

When you break your ankle, expecting it to heal 100% is probably not realistic. It's expected that your ankle may be weaker even after it heals and for symptoms to remain, even if it's just an ache in the winter. Knowing this, why would anyone think the brain would heal 100%? That's a high expectation for a squishy organ made up of delicate cells. Consequently, your brain may not ever recover to 100% of your previous self, and that's okay. In this book you will find ways to live with your head injury while getting to know the new you.

Keep in mind that recovery after a head injury can last from two weeks to several years. People can heal at varying rates, even if they suffer the same type of head injury. I often tell my patients that their brains will heal when they're ready to heal. But although there are things you can do to support your healing, you cannot speed up your brain's recovery. As expected, your brain really is the boss of you in this situation.

Nevertheless, most people recover from a mild head injury within two years.[2] After two years, your recovery may continue, but improvements in brain function will be subtle and incremental. Being older, female, and having had a previous head injury can increase your risk of a prolonged recovery.[3] Furthermore, a medical history of migraine headaches, depression, or anxiety are also thought to contribute to prolonged recovery periods.

During my first year of recovery, I saw a lot of improvement in my brain function and was able to return to work full time. In order to do this, however, there was a lot of sleeping involved, and I needed to learn to compensate for certain deficiencies like forgetfulness, lack of organization, and sensitivity to light and sound. I ended up developing several coping strategies and tools that I will share with you in this book.

Up to three years after my head injury, I continued to need a lot of sleep, but I was able to do a lot more during this time. I was able to slowly start exercising again and walking on my days off. It was during this time that I also decided to change careers, taking a bunch of continuing education courses in neurology and training under the neurologists that I worked with for three months. After two years, I worked more independently and

---

[2] Simon Fleminger and Jennie Ponsford, "Long-Term Outcome after Traumatic Brain Injury," *BMJ* 331 (December 15, 2005): 1419–20, https://doi.org/10.1136/bmj.331.7530.1419.

[3] Raaj Kishore Biswas, Enamul Kabir, and Rachel King, "Effect of Sex and Age on Traumatic Brain Injury: A Geographical Comparative Study," *Archives of Public Health* 75, no. 43, https://www.doi.org/10.1186/s13690-017-0211-y.

needed to consult with the neurologist less. I was doing better by this time but still had headaches most days, until they started to fade away four years after my car crash.

During the fifth year of recovery from my TBI, I started to write this book. I was able to do normal things again, like going to the movies and music concerts, and overall, I felt less overwhelmed by daily life. To this day I'm getting better though I'm still not 100%. I still have cognitive fatigue, sound sensitivity, light sensitivity, and difficulty with focus and concentration. I expect those things may never go away, but that's okay. I am certainly a different person than I was prior to my head injury, and I'm simply getting to know the new me.

Considering these facts, it's best to maintain realistic recovery expectations, allowing flexibility for setbacks and periods of regression in your recovery. A concussion is not like a cold, where you can anticipate feeling better in a few days.

While you wait for your brain to recover, it's best to look back at your progress and note your accomplishments. Don't focus on the future or worry about what you can't do now. Instead, focus on living in the moment and appreciating each day.

My head injury was the start of a new life and personal journey of self-rediscovery.

On a beautiful sunny day in April of 2016, I was out on my deck, talking to a friend on the phone. I told her about how I read everything I could on how to recover from a head injury. At the time, I was going on 20 years of working as a cardiology nurse practitioner. My friend suggested I go into neurology because she felt I would be a good patient advocate due to my head injury experience. This idea had not occurred to me until my friend brought it to my mind. I was so excited about the possibilities of changing my career to neurology that I couldn't sleep that night and ended up staying up late writing all the steps I needed to take to qualify for a job in this field. Two years later I was able to start a new job as a neurology nurse practitioner and have loved the career change ever since.

As a neurology nurse practitioner, I've had a front-row seat to patients coming in who struggle with many of the same things I struggled with when I went through my head injury. When speaking to my patients regarding their recovery, I also discovered they, too, were not aware of what was available to help them continue to work and study while they healed.

I've been there, done that, and got the T-shirt in my closet to prove it. My T-shirt says "My life went to hell in a handbasket, I made mistakes, but I survived." So, pull up a chair, grab a cup of coffee, and let's talk.

Section II

Symptoms

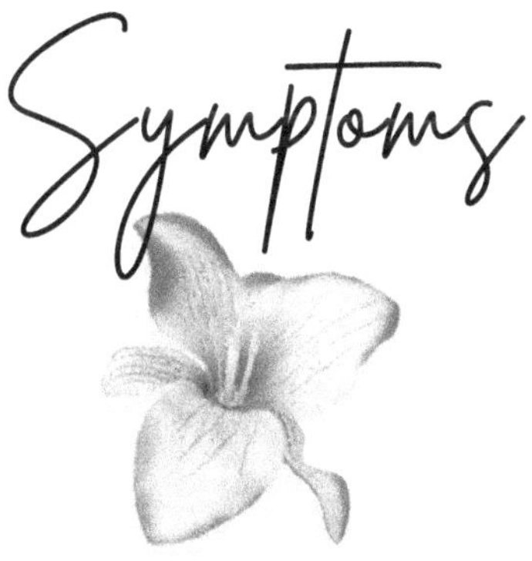

Chapter 2

Common Symptoms after a Head Injury

AFTER A HEAD INJURY, you may think you're going crazy as you cringe under fluorescent lights, wonder why the world around you is so loud, and can't seem to think or talk straight. There's a myriad of symptoms one can suffer after surviving a head injury, like short-term memory loss and sleep disturbance. However, there are other symptoms that run the gamut from physical to emotional and behavioral—all of which may affect your personal and professional life.

Waking up every morning day after day feeling tired, dizzy, and irritable and having a headache may seem like a nightmarish way to start your day. Unfortunately, after a head injury, this is simply how most mornings start. This is your new normal, as they say. Every day as you drag yourself out of bed, it's common to wonder if you will ever feel okay again.

Even if you're told by your doctor that you have a mild concussion, you will find that there's nothing mild about your head injury. You may feel as if you're going crazy as the life you knew before your head injury has been shattered, and the tiny shards are slowly scattering in the winds. Feeling lonely, being lost in your head, and wondering what's wrong with you as your mood swings and meager memory leave you confused and discombobulated are common too.

Attempting to get back into the swing of things at work or school may come with issues as well. There might be a significant change in your ability to focus, concentrate, think, and learn. You may find that the lights at work seem bright or ponder why everyone at school is talking so loudly. You may feel slow, unmotivated, and distracted as you toil to keep up with your workload. While it's possible to continue functioning enough to be at work or school, your work performance may often be way below what it was prior to your head injury. Because of this, you find yourself falling behind on deadlines or having to work long hours just to keep up.

When returning to school or work, you may feel as if you're slipping behind in your studies or barely holding down your job. What you're experiencing and going through is real. The truth is, there's nothing mild about a concussion or TBI. It's a serious game changer. But I promise there is hope.

Head injury symptoms can vary from mild to disabling. It's possible to have only one symptom or many symptoms. These can last for a couple weeks or for several years. Some symptoms will go away, and other new symptoms may pop up. Symptoms may overlap like colors in a kaleidoscope or trigger one another in a vicious tag team cycle. Sometimes, it may take you a few months to realize that you have head injury symptoms, because they were hidden under your other painful injuries.

The CDC lists the symptoms for mild TBI and concussion on their website.[4] The CDC further explains that they can vary from person to person and can change while you are recovering. Some of these symptoms are behavioral or physical changes—for example, changes in your vision, sound sensitivity, difficulty speaking, dizziness, headaches, and unrelenting fatigue.[5] Head injury symptoms can be life changing for some people and affect your ability to work or study.

---

[4] "Symptoms of Mild TBI and Concussion," Centers for Disease Control and Prevention, updated March 7, 2022, https://www.cdc.gov/traumaticbraininjury/concussion/symptoms.html.

[5] "Symptoms of Mild TBI and Concussion," Centers for Disease Control and Prevention.

Brainline.org reports that the CDC estimates that 2.8 million people in the United States sustain a TBI annually and that the cost in medical care and lost productivity in the U.S. was estimated to be $60 billion in 2000.[6] The CDC in 1999 reported that 5.3 million Americans were living with a permanent TBI–related disability.[7] While these statistics are alarming, research suggests that these numbers may be much higher, since they currently only account for people who are hospitalized.

SYMPTOMS YOU MAY HAVE

Although symptoms can vary from person to person, below are some of the common ailments that can affect you after suffering from a brain injury:

1. **Behavior changes:** Being irritable or becoming more tearful over the smallest things is common. Changes to your behavior or personality are one of the hardest consequences of a head injury to self-monitor and control.

2. **Vision changes:** A head injury can change how your eyes function or can damage the brain's visual processing abilities. This can cause blurred vision, difficulty with balance, dizziness, or changes in your ability to read. If you have similar symptoms, you should have your vision evaluated prior to returning to work or school.

3. **Hearing:** Trauma to the head can cause trouble with hearing related to sound sensitivity, hearing loss, vertigo, and tinnitus. These symptoms will make you want to avoid going out and participating in large social gatherings, cause fatigue, and make it difficult to concentrate at work or school.

---

[6] "Get the Stats on Traumatic Brain Injury in the United States," Brainline, April 27, 2017, https://www.brainline.org/article/get-stats-traumatic-brain-injury-united-states.

[7] Centers for Disease Control and Prevention, *Report to Congress: Traumatic Brain Injury in the United States*, December 1999, https://www.cdc.gov/traumaticbraininjury/pubs/tbi_report_to_congress.html.

4. **Speech:** Difficulty with finding words and struggling to say words are common symptoms of a head injury. These symptoms often worsen when you're tired, stressed, or distracted.

5. **Dizziness:** It's common for people to have dizziness after a head injury. These symptoms can last a couple weeks to several years. Dizziness can affect your ability to work on a computer, exercise, or drive. If you experience dizziness, you may need to see various specialists, from ear, nose, and throat doctors to behavioral optometrists, in order to figure out the cause of this symptom.

6. **Headache:** Headaches after a head injury can be mild to disabling. Headaches cause fatigue, irritability, and an inability to concentrate. These symptoms can also lead to missed days from work or school.

7. **Fatigue:** Fatigue is one of the most common and persistent symptoms after a head injury.[8] This type of fatigue is life-altering exhaustion that can come on after the slightest effort.

Many of these symptoms changed my life, and they still affect me now, even after I developed coping strategies. Here's just one example. Prior to my head injury, I would make notes when I would plan to speak during a work meeting. These days, preparing for a meeting is a big production for me.

First I plan to get nine to 10 hours of good sleep for a few nights prior to the meeting. I then spend several days gathering my thoughts, and I work on my talking points, with additional effort placed on screening out emotional issues. At the meeting, I practice deep breathing, reference my notes when speaking, and intentionally slow down my speech to ensure that my words come out clearly.

After the meeting I retreat to quickly write down what was discussed before I forget. For the rest of the day, I'm exhausted and unable to take on

---

[8] Kathleen R. Bell, "Fatigue and Traumatic Brain Injury," Model Systems Knowledge Translation Center, accessed April 18, 2022, https://msktc.org/tbi/factsheets/fatigue-and-traumatic-brain-injury.

complicated tasks. If the meeting is intense and stressful, I end up missing the next two to three days of work. It's not uncommon to sleep 12 hours a night in order to replenish my cognitive energy and restore my emotional control.

These symptoms can blur into each other or sneak up on you like falling dominos, as one symptom triggers another. In the next chapters, I will go into more detail regarding the above symptoms and the specialists who can help you cope while you wait for your brain to heal.

Chapter 3

Vision A Not-So-Fun Fun House

W HEN MY KIDS WERE younger, we used to love to run through carnival fun houses together. We would laugh at our distorted images in the mirrors, blink at the flashing, bright lights, and giggle as we struggled not to fall while walking over spinning roller pins, shifting floors, and a tumbling, turning tunnel.

Fun houses are delightful to visit, but no one would ever want to live in one. That's sort of what life is like after a brain injury. I've lived in one for many years. Sometimes, it feels as if I were surrounded by mirrors, and I don't know which way to walk without running into one.

Disruption to your brain's intricate ability to process your vision can result in a multitude of symptoms. In her book, *Mild Traumatic Brain Injury: The Guidebook,* Mary Lou Acimovic refers to this as post-traumatic vision syndrome.[9]

After a head injury, some people may lose their peripheral vision or

---

[9] Mary Lou Acimovic, *Mild Traumatic Brain Injury: The Guidebook* (self-published, 2010), 38.

have blurred vision or double vision. It may be difficult to notice because the change might be slight.

While reading for a duration of time your vision might blur. You may have difficulty focusing your eyes on objects, or you may notice your focus is slow to change when moving from near to far objects. You might also notice your eyes lose focus or feel strained, or have pain behind the eyes, after looking at a computer screen for a certain amount of time.

There are some symptoms you may be surprised are caused by a problem with your vision. These symptoms can consist of things like mild to severe headaches, cognitive fatigue with reading, or decreased tolerance to prolonged work on a computer. Some people may even suffer from anxiety, dizziness, and difficulty with balance.

Difficulty finding objects, such as a bottle of spice or a bag of beans on the grocery shelf, are other common symptoms you may or may not notice. Dizziness or nausea while following a moving object with your eyes might occur frequently as well.

Photophobia, which is sensitivity to light or bright lights, is possible. I have also had patients report seeing an annoying intermittent glare after their head injury. This is why it's important to have your vision evaluated by a TBI vision specialist following an incident. One type of specialist is a behavioral optometrist. These specialists often belong to the Neuro-Optometric Rehabilitation Association.

THE EYES ARE THE WINDOW TO YOUR BRAIN

The ability to see the things in the world around you is a complex process that's managed by the coordinated work of your eyes and brain. There are several areas in the brain that play a part in visual perception and processing. This information is too overwhelming to share in just one book, and my intentions here are not to give you a headache. I just want to point out a few parts of this amazing, complex, and intricate process.

The eyes are the window to your brain. They communicate the information of images they see by displaying it onto your retina, the back wall of your eye. A delicate nerve called the optic nerve then transmits this information to the back part of your brain called the occipital lobes. This is where your visual cortex resides, which receives input from the retina and the optic nerve.

This being said, you can see how easy it would be to knock this complicated process off-line with just the right blow.

One of my patients suffered a strike to the back of the head. After his injury he reported having dizziness when tracking objects, while working on the computer, and when watching action movies on the TV. Scrolling up or down on the computer or his smartphone caused him to feel nauseous. For a while he could not drive because the movement of the car made him dizzy, and when he was a passenger in the car, he had to look down to prevent getting carsick. Fortunately, with time and treatment, his symptoms resolved.

Another one of my patients was in a motor vehicle accident and struck the side of her head on the driver's side window. She had several common post-concussion symptoms, such as headaches, light sensitivity, difficulty with her memory, and irritability, and she reported seeing an annoying intermittent glare in her peripheral vision. This glaring light would worsen while she was driving or outside. Wearing hats and sunglasses helped, and over time and with constant management of her post-concussion headaches, the glaring light lessened, and she was able to return to driving.

In their book, *Coping with Concussion and Mild Traumatic Brain Injury: A Guide to Living with Challenges Associated with Post Concussion Syndrome and Brain Trauma*, Dr. Diane Stoler and Barbara Hill explain that an "injury to the crown area (the top of the head) can affect the parietal lobes, which governs spatial awareness and higher-level visual skills such as reading."[10]

A disruption to any of these delicate tissues may affect your visual cognition and visual perception speed. These damaged areas in your brain's visual processing will affect the speed with which your eyes move to focus and perceive what's in front of them along with your brain's ability to process and accurately interpret the information your eyes are sending.

You're Not Crazy—You Just Can't See Straight

Seeing a specialist will help identify issues you may be having with vision. It will be a relief to know you're not going crazy and that there's a physical cause and treatment for your symptoms. Here's a list of the most misdiagnosed vision problems:

- Vision overstimulation
- Blurred vision
- Double vision
- Binocular vision dysfunction

A traditional eye exam looks at and measures eye acuity, which is how your eyes see. Measuring eye acuity tells your provider the clarity or sharpness of your vision. These exams determine how well you see the detail of objects close and far away. However, this does not evaluate how well your eyes work together when you attempt to focus on an object or view.

These providers will often tell you after a head injury that your eyes are healthy or that your prescription has not changed. If you've injured your brain and would like to see a specialist, consider making an appointment with an optometrist, an ophthalmologist, a behavioral optometrist, a neuro-optometrist, or a neuro–physical therapist.

---

[10] Diane Stoler and Barbara Hill, *Coping with Concussion and Mild Traumatic Brain Injury: A Guide to Living with Challenges Associated with Post Concussion Syndrome and Brain Trauma* (New York: Avery, 2013), 135.

Optometrists, behavioral optometrists, and neuro-optometrists usually do not require a referral in order to make an appointment to see them. Specialists such as the ophthalmologist or neuro–physical therapist require a referral from your general practitioner. If your doctor, despite the request for the referral based on your symptoms you have presented, is not willing to provide a referral, then you should say you are insisting on the referral or that your family is concerned and requesting the referral. If your general practitioner still refuses to provide you a referral, I recommend you fire them and get a more understanding primary care provider.

Ophthalmologists screen for diplopia, also known as double vision. If you have diplopia, these doctors can provide you with prism glasses to help correct your double vision.

A behavioral optometry exam shows how well your brain's visual process is working. Behavioral optometrists specialize in identifying small misalignments caused by disruptions in your brain's visual process. Behavioral optometrists look for problems with your eye movement and issues with the eyes moving together for tracking, and they check how well the eyes work together to pick up environmental information. These visual misalignments drain energy from the brain and can worsen other symptoms.

A neuro-physical therapist can help identify issues with the eyes' ability to track objects and can treat symptoms such as dizziness. Ideally your vision evaluation should be completed and treated prior to you returning to work or school. Also keep in mind that, as your brain heals, your vision may change. If this is the case, you'll need to follow up with your eye specialist for adjustments in your therapy.

Vision Influences Perception

Having your vision evaluated and treated can be an effective way to reduce headaches and anxiety after a brain injury. Not getting these issues identified and treated can lead to a longer and more miserable recovery.

Undiagnosed post-traumatic vision syndrome can be irritating at the very least, although for others, it can be so disabling that the person is unable to read, drive, or exercise. How quickly these symptoms resolve depends on how hard you hit your head, the type of injury your brain sustained, if your eye was directly affected by the impact, and the location in the brain where the injury occurred.

With time, appropriate treatment, and therapy, most people will recover their baseline vision, or at least see (pun intended) a significant improvement with their vision.

TYPES OF ISSUES

There are many issues that can affect your vision after a head injury. Therefore, an evaluation by the appropriate specialist will be needed. I had two visual issues after my head injury. One was visual overstimulation, and the other was binocular vision dysfunction (BVD).

A person with visual overstimulation after a head injury cannot tolerate changing light patterns, the sight of movement, or clutter. A person with visual overstimulation may be mildly bothered or completely incapacitated by these symptoms.

For me this felt like being in a fun house hallway of mirrors with strobe lights and not knowing which way to step without face-planting into a mirror. I found myself succumbing to apathy, trapped between a cluttered kitchen countertop and a dining room table strewn with paperwork and coffee cups.

Once you're diagnosed with visual overstimulation, caring for this symptom involves getting your home and work environment organized.

BINOCULAR VISION DYSFUNCTION (BVD)

After a head injury, BVD is a commonly missed diagnosis. The Vision Specialists of Michigan estimate that vertical heterophoria, a form of BVD, may affect 50% of people who have persistent symptoms after a head injury.[11] Some of the symptoms of BVD are, but are not limited to, headaches, migraines, dizziness, nausea, head "tilting" toward one shoulder, closing one eye to read, light sensitivity, blurred or double vision, neck pain, difficulty with balance, coordination, reading, and concentrating.[12]

For me, this was the turning, tumbling tunnel in the fun house. My balance felt off, as if I were being pulled to the right, the way you are in the tunnel. I had headaches and neck pain because I was tilting my head to the right and straining my eyes to help clear up my vision. As well, when I walked, I had to watch the ground to keep myself from losing my balance.

If you're referred to a behavioral optometrist, plan for the exam to be extensive, sometimes lasting two to four hours. Once your exam is completed, you will be prescribed glasses to correct your misalignment. The optometrist will want you to return three to six months after wearing your corrective glasses to see if your eyes' misalignment has changed. This can happen after wearing your prescription glasses, which helps your eye muscles relax.

My glasses helped improve my walking and balance. I could walk straighter and look up at my surroundings, which felt like a luxury. My new glasses increased my cognitive stamina as well, allowing me to read and work on the computer longer. There was no longer a perceptual delay in my eyes' ability to change focus. My neck pain went away because I was no longer having to tilt my head to the right to see. My headaches decreased over time, and it's to the point now that I rarely get a headache.

For me this diagnosis and treatment was a miracle. I was able to improve my performance at work and have leftover energy to enjoy my weekends. I was able to stop living in a not-so-fun fun house.

---

[11] "Michigan Eye Specialists Helps Veterans Suffering from TBI," Vision Specialists of Michigan, October 10, 2013, https://www.vision-specialists.com/press/veteran-connect-october-10-2013/.

[12] "Binocular Vision Dysfunction Symptoms," Vision Specialists of Michigan, accessed April 14, 2022, https://www.vision-specialists.com/binocular-vision-dysfunction/symptoms/.

Chapter 4

Hearing It's a Loud, Loud, Loud, Loud World

WITHOUT THINKING ABOUT IT, early into my recovery I stopped listening to music in my car. When I listened to music, I would start to feel drowsy. Music also hurt my ears and gave me headaches. At first, I didn't make the connection between music and my fatigue and headaches.

I remember being at work and wondering why everyone was always talking so *loudly*. I found myself being distracted by conversations outside my office in a way that I had not noticed before my head injury.

Before my head injury, my husband and I would catch up with each other at the end of the day while watching the news. After my head injury, my poor husband learned the hard way not to attempt to have a conversation with me while the TV volume was on. First I would struggle to understand what he was talking about. Then after a while, I would get irritable and impatient every time he started talking. He quickly found that he was able to keep his head from being torn off if he put the TV on mute or paused it before he started to talk to me.

When I was at work, I felt tired and irritable and struggled to focus. Using my noise-canceling headphones often kept me from breaking down in tears. After my head injury, the world was just too loud for me. My sound sensitivity limited my social life and ended my ability to attend music concerts and see movies in a theater.

Don't Miss Out on Life

Trauma to your head can cause havoc to your hearing and your brain's ability to process what it hears in the environment. A head injury can lead to a multitude of hearing problems and symptoms. At the very least, these symptoms can be annoying. At the worst, they can be disabling.

This is why it's important to get your hearing evaluated by a specialist if you start experiencing any symptoms. Not getting your hearing symptoms evaluated may lead you to feeling overwhelmed and anxious in noisy environments, which can make you avoid engaging in some of your favorite activities. Hearing issues can make you feel isolated and alone—for example, if you're unable to hear telephone conversations or to focus on a conversation while out with your friends. Untreated hearing symptoms may affect your performance at work and your ability to learn in school.

However, before you go to see a specialist, it's important to know what the symptoms are so that you can effectively describe them. Your hearing symptoms are not like a rash or a fever that a doctor can visibly detect. They are something that only you can experience and attempt to describe.

Here are some of the common hearing symptoms caused by head injuries:

- Sound sensitivity, also known as hyperacusis
- Hearing loss
- Vertigo or dizziness
- Feeling off balanced
- Feeling fullness in the ear

- Tinnitus
- Difficulty with your hearing or with understanding conversations
- Feeling overwhelmed and anxious when out in noisy environments
- Feeling fatigued after being in a noisy environment

If you think you may have sensitivity to sound, you should fill out a Khalfa Hyperacusis questionnaire.[13] It's a tool that screens for hyperacusis. It will tell you and your doctor your level of sensitivity to sounds.

If you have issues with your hearing, you should be evaluated by a specialist. Sometimes, your symptoms are not just something to deal with. On occasion these symptoms are indicators that there's an underlying issue that can be treated.

HEARING SYMPTOMS

A rare symptom after a head injury is hyperacusis, also known as sound hypersensitivity. "Hyperacusis is a reduction of normal tolerances for everyday sounds," say H. Silverstein, J. Smith and B. Kellermeyer in their article in *American Journal of Otolaryngology*.[14] Hyperacusis can be due to an inner ear injury in the auditory system, which can make it sensitive to noise.

Another auditory symptom that can occur after a concussion is hearing overload. Dr. Diane Stoler and Barbara Hill, in their book, *Coping with Concussion and Mild Traumatic Brain Injury*, explain that "hearing overload can cause sounds to be magnified or make it difficult to understand conversations in a noisy room."[15] What happens after a head injury is that the brain is unable to filter out background noise, making it difficult to

---

[13] Khalfa et al., "Modified Khalfa Hyperacusis Questionnaire," Tinnitus Practitioners Association, 2002, http://kytinnitustreatment.com/wp-content/uploads/2015/06/TPA-Khalfa-Hyperacusis-Questionaire.pdf.

[14] Herbert Silverstein, Joshua Smith, and Brian Kellermeyer, "Stapes Hypermobility as a Possible Cause of Hyperacusis," *American Journal of Otolaryngology* 40, no. 2 (March–April 2019): 247, https://doi.org/10.1016/j.amjoto.2018.10.018.

[15] Stoler and Hill, *Coping with Concussion*, 209.

interpret and differentiate sounds in the environment. This can make you feel overwhelmed or anxious if you're in a loud restaurant or bar—or if your husband is trying to talk to you while you're watching TV.

Another common symptom is tinnitus. Tinnitus is a ringing or buzzing noise in the ear that can occur after a head injury. Sometimes this symptom is described as a hissing, high-pitch ringing, or a roaring sound. These sounds worsen when you're in a quiet space or at night when you're trying to sleep.

I also developed tinnitus after my head injury, so not only is the world now too loud, but it also does not shut up, even when I am trying to sleep.

In addition to my hearing symptoms, I also had difficulty with my balance. This is when I found out about superior semicircular canal dehiscence (SSCD). Sounds scary, right? That's because it is.

SSCD can happen with head trauma. It's when a blow to the head causes a breach in the overlying bone that's supposed to cover the superior semicircular canal. This overlying bone protects this sensitive organ from exposure to external sound and pressure. The superior semicircular canal is in the inner ear and is responsible for communicating the rotational movement of your head to your brain. People with SSCD can have sensitivity to loud sounds and report that they can hear their eyes move or that their voices sound too loud. Loud noise from the environment, or even a cough, may cause objects to move in their vision. Other symptoms include difficulty with balance and disequilibrium. A specialist can order a CT scan to screen for SSCD.

After seeing a behavioral optometrist, it was noted that when I wore noise-canceling headphones, my walking improved. My doctor told me about SSCD and had me complete a head CT scan that specifically looked for SSCD. Fortunately, my CT scan came back negative.

With hyperacusis, there's an argument that the use of sound-filtering tools leads to becoming desensitized to noise. Dr. Nigel King speaks to this in his book, *Overcoming Mild Traumatic Brain Injury and Post-Concussion*

Symptoms: A Self-Help Guide Using Evidence-Based Techniques, stating that "using earplugs or hearing protection, however, are not usually good long-term strategies."[16] He goes on to say that desensitization is the preferred treatment for many who have suffered a head injury and are sensitive to sounds.[17]

However, there's plenty of controversy surrounding the treatment of sound sensitivity. While some therapists believe sound-filtering equipment should be employed to help improve quality of life, others warn against overuse of noise-canceling technology or earplugs.[18] Such therapists argue that sound-filtering equipment will only make the symptoms worse by exposing the ear to prolonged periods of protection from sound. Yet, the therapists who advocate for the use of sound-filtering devices point out that there's not enough research to support this belief. I say do what works best for you.

Over time as my brain healed, I was able to tolerate more noise. I slowly needed to use my sound-filtering tools less at home. However, at work I still use my sound-filtering tools when I need to apply my brain energy to focus and concentrate on my work. I have also used them when I go to the theater or when I find myself in a loud restaurant.

I would recommend listening to the world when you can. "Current studies show that filters can reduce overstimulation to the auditory system and allow you to participate in social situations without becoming overwhelmed," say Dr. Mary Keatley and Laura Whittemore in their book, *Recovering from Mild Traumatic Brain Injury (MTBI): A Handbook of Hope for Our Military Warriors and Their Families*.[19] When you start to feel stressed, fatigued, or dizzy, or when you get a headache, seek a quiet place

---

[16] Nigel S. King, *Overcoming Mild Traumatic Brain Injury and Post-Concussion Symptoms: A Self-Help Guide Using Evidence-Based Techniques* (London: Robinson, 2015), 146.

[17] King, *Overcoming Mild Traumatic Brain Injury*, 146.

[18] Mary Ann Keatley and Laura L. Whittemore, *Recovering from Mild Traumatic Brain Injury (MTBI): A Handbook of Hope for Our Military Warriors and Their Families* (Littleton, CO: Brain Injury Hope Foundation, 2009), 18-19.

[19] Keatley and Whittemore, *Recovering from Mild Traumatic Brain Injury*, 19.

or use your noise-filtering tools.

Again, it comes down to what works for you. You will need to find the balance between protecting your brain's healing energy and challenging your brain to grow stronger.

GETTING ANSWERS

If you have any of the above-listed hearing symptoms or experience difficulty hearing, focusing, or concentrating, you should seek an evaluation from a specialist. When you meet with the specialist, ask if they have experience in treating patients with head injuries. Once your hearing issue is diagnosed, you can either get it treated or implement strategies that will help you cope with the symptoms as you wait for your brain to heal. This will help save your brain energy.

Ask your doctor for a referral to a specialist. Some of these specialists include audiologists and otolaryngologists, which are also known as ear, nose, and throat specialists. An audiologist can also do a test called loudness discomfort level.

Fortunately, most hearing issues from head injuries heal with time. See your doctor about getting your hearing evaluated by a hearing specialist. Get the care your brain needs to support its healing so you can keep working or studying and get back to living your life to the fullest.

Chapter 5

Communication Breakdown
Star Trek versus Starbucks

IT WAS THE DAY after my car accident, and I was back at work. I had a slight headache and felt tired and achy, but I just chalked that up to being in a crash. I hadn't yet been diagnosed with any sort of brain trauma. At midday, my nursing colleagues and I decided to take a break from a meeting and go grab some coffee. "Let's go get some *Star Trek*," I proposed.

My colleagues stopped and looked at me. One cocked her head and asked, "What did you just say?"

"I meant to say, 'Let's go get some Starbucks,' " I said. "What did I just say?"

Shaking her head, she said, "You said '*Star Trek.*' "

My highly protective colleagues promptly told me I had probably sustained a concussion and needed to see my doctor as soon as possible.

I was unaware of any changes in my behavior, but my friend pointed out on our drive home that I had not been acting normally. She made me promise to see my doctor the next day. I did, and they were right. It wouldn't be the first time I would mix things up. *Star Trek*, by the way, doesn't go well with coffee.

Oh, Crap, What Was I Saying?

Struggling with words, both finding and saying them, is a common complaint of patients who have suffered a head injury. You know how you scramble for a word and are frustrated when you can't find it? People with head injuries feel that way every day.

When you have a brain injury, your biggest fear is losing your job or failing in school, because you are seen as incompetent. The last thing you want is for people to think you're dim-witted. Making written mistakes or struggling to find your words in front of others is embarrassing. It exacerbates these understandable worst fears and can add to your already heightened anxiety.

It's as if my brain just sits back and laughs as it makes me look like a dullard spouting off malapropisms in a Shakespearean play. Ugh! Complete humiliation nation!

Common Communication Symptoms

Feeling stressed, anxious, upset, or tired will make it even harder to find the word you want. Being able to find and say words is a higher executive function that requires a lot of cognitive energy. After a head injury, these brain functions are glitchy at best and often run on sloth mode. As a result, you may notice some of these symptoms:

- Difficulty finding a word
- Feeling like your speech is slow
- Running words together
- When you think of one word but say another word

- Inability to say words correctly and clearly
- Increase in typos or spelling errors
- Difficulty with handwriting

Just Laugh It Off

The first thing to remember is that people with healthy brains also make mistakes, lose their train of thought, and flounder to find their words. They also send emails with typos and misspelled words. They also say *"Star Trek"* instead of "Starbucks."

If you're like me and do not want to reveal to others that you're recovering from a brain injury, you can gloss over these moments with humor.

When I find myself floundering to speak, I distract others by saying, "Oh man, I need more coffee," or "You know, you are talking to a blond," or "Oops, senior moment." Feel free to use these phrases or make up your own.

So don't panic when these issues spring up. Instead, embrace learning to laugh at your tongue-tied moments. Keeping company with a good sense of self-deprecating humor will take the edge off your worries, embarrassment, and fears.

Where in the Word

My favorite thing to do is send off a work email that I proofread multiple times only to find typos or words that sound alike but mean different things. Ugh, not!

You may have difficulty with spelling or sounding words out, or you might substitute words that sound the same, or see yourself writing down the wrong word.

There may be times that a co-worker or instructor will point out a mistake you made. Try not to get defensive. You should respond with "Thank you for pointing this out," or "Thank you for bringing this to my attention." This is not an easy automatic response when you're struck with fear or embarrassment. You may feel you have been caught making a mistake. If needed, practice saying this response with family and friends so it's automatic when you're at work or school.

Then, if possible, correct the mistake and try not to make the same mistake again. (I share some tips below on how to do this.) Owning up to a mistake and being willing to correct it goes a long way in maintaining your credibility and positive relationships with others. We all know that no one likes a person when they deny errors, blame others, or make excuses for their mistakes.

If someone points out one of your mistakes in jest and teases you about it, just laugh with them and then walk away. Some people are just trying to inject humor into their workday, while others might be trying to make themselves feel better at your expense. What you don't want to do is panic, get frustrated, or become defensive. These people are not worth your precious brain energy.

REBOOTING YOUR SYSTEM

Every day, even today, my brain blanks out on words and my tongue trips into tangles. After a head injury, the brain's language centers are kicked off-line, and connections between neurons are lost. You need to start reconnecting and rebooting the system. Over time I have learned some tips and tricks that have helped me clear out my cognitive carburetor.

To get my brain's bundled-up wires going in the morning, I write in my journal. The act of handwriting for me seems to help clear out the morning fog in my brain and to reconnect my brain to my body. As I write I feel my mental clarity increase, and I see and feel my difficulty to draw letters improve as I write two to three sentences. Maybe daily handwriting will help you and your brain too.

Speaking, listening, and reading are three separate but overlapping activities that require the brain's language centers. If one of them goes off-line or is cluttered with gunk, you can use another to provide assistance or backup. For instance, one thing I do is practice saying words and people's names out loud several times. I do this before speaking to others. Another trick I use is to write down words I have difficulty saying before meeting with the person I am going to speak to. For me, seeing a word helps me say it and recall it more easily.

The other tool you can use is sending emails. For some people, after a head injury, it's easier to communicate through written words rather than over the phone. Writing things down not only helps you remember but also gives you a place to store important information.

If you struggle with speaking, simply slowing down the pace of your speech may help. You can also practice saying the words you wish to speak by writing down words and sounding them out slowly and deliberately.

Speak to a Specialist

If after your head injury you note difficulty in your verbal or written communication, ask your primary care doctor for a referral to a specialist. Some of these specialists are neurologists or speech and language pathologists, also known as speech therapists. You can also ask for a referral to have a neuropsychological assessment. These specialists can pinpoint your language or speech issues and recommend treatment and therapies.

Remember that you're still smart—you and your brain are healing. With time you and your brain will develop new pathway connections and strategies to promote a better brain performance when it comes to communicating your words. Until then, learn to laugh at yourself and your brain while enjoying a cup of *Star Trek*—I mean, Starbucks—coffee.

Chapter 6

Dizziness I'm Not Drunk!

MY NEIGHBORS PROBABLY THINK I'm an alcoholic. I'm not. I just occasionally fall while taking out the trash cans, lose my balance while planting flowers, and stumble and sway as I walk down my driveway. When I fall in my front yard after crouching down to pick weeds, I just want to jump up with my hands in the air and yell, "I'm not drunk; I just have a brain injury!"

Sometimes I feel as if I've moved permanently onto a party boat where I'm left to feel out of sorts, stumbling around as I yell in my head, "I am not drunk; I'm just dizzy."

For you, these symptoms may come and go, while for others, their symptoms will be persistent. These symptoms for you may be annoying or disabling. The severity of these symptoms depends on the type and seriousness of your brain injury. Other injuries to your neck, ears, eyes, legs, or feet will compound your symptoms. For some people these symptoms can persist for years.

My dizziness accompanies emotional stress and fatigue. Sometimes I will turn in bed and feel as if I were on a rollercoaster. At other times when I'm sitting still, the world will feel as if it were moving without me. When I'm tired and not paying attention, I can lose my balance and fall when I move too fast.

Thank goodness many years of training in martial arts has taught me how to fall.

Some people will have dizziness every time they turn their head fast. Others will experience dizziness when tracking moving objects with their eyes. People report feeling unsteady with walking or a sense of disconnection with their feet. Many head injury patients have even said they will feel lightheaded while in a grocery store or loud environment. Head injury specialists believe this is due to sensory overload.

The origin of these symptoms can be difficult to figure out because many areas of the brain and the systems it uses to process information can be affected. Your brain is told where you are in space through many sensory avenues that include your vision, balance organs in your inner ear, and the receptors in your neck and feet. Also, injuries to the back of your head and neck can cause damage to your brain stem and cerebellum where your brain controls balance and movement.

Prior to your head injury, all these systems work in sequence. After a head injury, these systems' connections have been knocked off-line. These systems may even compete for your brain's attention instead of providing the brain with a unifying stream of information.

Don't forget these systems also need a lot of energy to run smoothly. This is energy your brain is not willing to share when it's in recovery.

Symptoms of dizziness after a head injury can be difficult to diagnose and manage—meaning you may need to prepare for a prolonged, problematic recovery from these types of post–head injury symptoms.

SYMPTOMS TO REPORT TO YOUR
BRAIN INJURY SPECIALIST

- Dizziness
- Lightheadedness
- Feeling disoriented
- Sensation of floating, not feeling grounded
- Vertigo
- Problems with balance
- Problems with coordination
- Feeling unsteady
- Bumping into people or objects
- Disequilibrium

PLEASE DON'T ROCK THE BOAT

Experts say most people will see their dizziness resolve in six to eight weeks after their head injury. This was not the case for me. My symptoms persisted for several years after my head injury. If you find yourself in the same rocking party boat with me, you may also notice that when you have a headache, feel stressed, or have not gotten enough sleep, these symptoms will return or worsen.

When you're dizzy, take it easy. You should avoid driving and high-impact exercise until your symptoms resolve. Feeling off-balance or dizzy can increase your risk of falling. The last thing you want is to fall and hit your head again or break a bone. I've seen this happen to some of my patients, leaving them with injuries, mental distress, anxiety, and fear of falling again.

I NEED HELP OFF THIS PARTY BOAT

A lot of people with head trauma and dizziness think they should be under the care of a neurologist. If you choose to see a neurologist, make sure you ask them if they specialize in head injury care. Most neurologists are general neurology providers, which means they specialize in treating diseases of the brain, like Parkinson's disease, epilepsy, and multiple sclerosis, which won't be of much help to you.

When I saw a neurologist, he ordered an MRI of my brain and provided me with a diagnosis of having a mild TBI. These were things I needed, but I wasn't provided with help in recovering from my brain injury. He just told me there was nothing he could do and to give myself some recovery time, which I've heard other neurologists tell patients.

I did not find this advice helpful. I could not wait at home to heal from my injury. What I needed was help getting back to work and life. Looking back, I realized I was asking for help from the wrong provider.

CHECK WITH YOUR DOCTOR

It's always a good idea to check in with your doctor, who can do a basic workup into your symptoms. Many medications, such as blood pressure medications and anti-seizure medications, can cause dizziness. Talk to your doctor about the benefit of continuing any medications that are making your symptoms worse. Often lowering your medication dose can be helpful.

Your doctor can also evaluate if you have orthostatic hypotension. This occurs when your blood pressure drops when you sit up in bed or stand from a chair. This drop in your blood pressure can cause dizziness and make you feel weak or unsteady on your feet.

Also ask for a referral to a specialist, preferably one who is experienced in treating patients with head injuries. Some of these specialists are neurotherapist, occupational therapists, physical therapists, and physical medicine and rehabilitation doctors (PM&R).

Neurotherapist

Neurotherapist will perform a comprehensive evaluation to see if your dizziness is from your inner ear or visual tracking issues and to determine whether you need help with walking and balance. They're physical therapists who train to help people with injuries to the central nervous system, which includes the brain and spinal cord. Their therapies will help treat your dizziness and help you regain your balance.

I loved my neurotherapist. I found her to be a wealth of helpful information. Unlike some ER doctors and general practitioners, she was sympathetic to my condition. She understood that I needed to get control of my symptoms so I could feel confident getting back to my job. She was aware of how little brain energy I had to spare on her therapies and encouraged me to work on my exercises when I had the energy and discouraged me from pushing myself too hard.

She determined that my dizziness was not vertigo related to benign paroxysmal positional vertigo (BPPV). BPPV can develop after a head injury due to tiny calcium particles that are knocked loose and moved from their normal place in the inner ear. These particles move with gravity. If they're not where they are supposed to be, they send your brain misinformation regarding the placement of your head. This misinformation can make the world feel as if it were spinning around you, which can make it difficult to stay balanced. If you have BPPV, a neurotherapist can help treat your symptoms.

My neurotherapist was able to pinpoint the source of my dizziness as the tracking of objects with my eyes. She taught me gaze exercises to help improve my visual processing speed, plus other exercises to help with my balance.

Occupational Therapist (OT)

Occupational therapists aid recovery from a brain injury by using everyday activities for therapy. This is accomplished by helping you maintain and recover function of daily living activities. They can evaluate your balance, coordination, and difficulties walking, then recommend assistive devices to help you prevent falls or other accidents.

Although I had symptoms of dizziness and often felt off-balance, I didn't need to go to an OT. However, I have referred several patients to OTs if they continue to have episodes of falling after seeing their physical therapist or neurotherapist. The benefit of an OT is that you can also have them come to your home and identify areas that increase your risk of a fall. The occupational therapist will provide you with recommendations to help create a safer home environment.

Physical Therapist (PT)

A physical therapist will help you heal from injuries sustained along with your head injury while also helping improve your movement and pain control of injured joints and muscles.

During my car accident, I sustained whiplash along with my head injury. Healing a neck injury helps with pain control, but it also helps with balance. There are receptors in the neck muscles that communicate to the brain the position of your head. These receptors get damaged when neck muscles are strained or torn. Your PT can help these muscles heal, which in turn will help your neck receptors better communicate information relating to where your head is in the world, keeping you balanced.

Physical Medicine and Rehabilitation Doctor (PM&R)

A PM&R doctor is also known as a physiatrist. They specialize in injuries that affect the brain, spine, muscles, and joints. A physiatrist can determine the extent of your head injury and assist with pain management from any other injuries you may have sustained. They also can refer you to other specialists as needed.

My physiatrist was amazing. She was the first doctor who recognized my symptoms. She was much more knowledgeable regarding head injuries than my primary care doctor and brought to light how my slow thinking process and cognitive fatigue were related to my concussion.

She was also the first doctor who explained to me that I needed to take time off from work so I could rest and begin the recovery process.

Fortunately, she took my injuries seriously and put me on the right track toward healing my head injury. Her interventions saved my life and my job.

SEE A SPECIALIST

Dizziness is difficult to diagnose and treat in patients with healthy brains. It's even more difficult when treating dizziness after a head injury. Unfortunately, there's not much a general practitioner or ER doctor can do to help you. There are simply too many variables at play when it comes to the brain, and they're not trained to know all of them. This is why it's important to track your symptoms so you can communicate them to your family doctor so they can make a recommendation to see a specialist. Your sense of dizziness could be due to multiple systems not working well after your head injury. So, it's reasonable that it may take multiple specialists to help you with your symptoms. With their guidance, they may be able to help you and your brain off the party boat.

Chapter 7

Headaches Living with Torture

Headaches are torture. When I say headaches, I mean the kind that feel as if your head were in the hands of a cruel master of torture. After my head injury, my torturer would put my head on a shelf with an ice pick through my right eye. Other days, the torturer would impale the back of my head onto a searing-hot spike. When she was feeling kind, she simply put my head into a vice.

I was in this torturer's hands for at least four years. The first two years were intense, but as time passed, she must have gotten bored and moved onto some other poor soul. Thankfully, I rarely draw her attention anymore.

Before my head injury, I was used to dealing with migraine headaches, but they were nothing compared to the pain of my post-traumatic headaches.

Post-Traumatic Headaches

Headaches after a head injury, also known as post-traumatic headaches, can be mild to downright disabling. If you're lucky, you may only have headaches for a couple weeks, but some people might have headaches for years after their head injury.

Your headaches after your head injury may feel different. Pain from a headache may change in location, and the type of pain can change from a mild ache to a stabbing, pounding, or burning pain. The intensity can also range from mild to severe, and the number of headaches you have in a month may increase as well.

This highlights why it's important to get control of your headaches, as severe pain drains energy, worsens cognitive functions, and can have an adverse effect on your mood. This can affect your work and school performance and lead to missed days in the office or classroom.

There are multiple types of post-traumatic headaches. Sometimes the type of head injury you experience, whether a blunt force trauma or blast injury, will increase your risk of certain types of post-traumatic headaches. Here's a brief list of common headaches and symptoms you may experience after a head injury:

- **Tension headache:** Generally you will feel as if there were a tight band around your head.
- **Migraine headache:** This type of headache usually causes pounding, pulsing, or throbbing pain on one side of the head and sometimes can cause stomach upset.
- **Occipital neuralgia:** This can cause severe sharp, throbbing, or shock-like pain that starts in your upper neck and can radiate to the back of your head or ear. It's usually caused by injury to a nerve that is under your scalp. This nerve can be injured, for example, during a whiplash injury to your neck.
- **Cluster headaches:** As their name implies, these headaches occur in groups or cyclic patterns. This type of headache is considered one the most painful headaches and often will wake you up in the middle of the night with severe, quick pain in or around one eye.

Rebound Headaches

The last thing you want is what is known as a rebound headache. Rebound headaches are awful and result from taking large amounts of over-the-counter or prescription pain medications. This creates a situation in which your body gets dependent on having these medications to keep you free of headaches, but the minute the medication clears out of your system, your headache returns. Some of these medications are aspirin, ibuprofen, acetaminophen, and caffeine. Yes, caffeine is not just for coffee—it's also a pain reliever found in some over-the-counter headache medications.

The treatment for rebound headaches is stopping all your pain medications for a minimum of three months. That also means no coffee or chocolate for three months too. This wash-out period can be difficult to get through and should be done under the supervision of your general health care provider or a headache specialist.

No One Likes a Pain in the Neck

When you sustain a head injury, your neck can be injured as well. That's why it's important to get your neck evaluated and treated, especially if you're in pain. Often neck pain can trigger headaches in many people with healthy brains. So, if your neck is not cared for, it will be difficult to control your headaches.

Luckily, there are many therapists who can assist you in controlling your neck pain while you wait for it to heal. One option is to see a PT, who will help treat your injured muscles with stretching, strengthening, and massage techniques. A PT will also give you tools for adjusting your posture and decreasing the weight-bearing load on your neck.

You can also see an acupuncturist or a massage therapist, who will help relieve muscle pain, reduce soreness, and offer prevention for future headaches. An acupuncturist uses very thin needles and places them in the skin in strategic spots to improve the flow of energy through your body. Acupuncture has been found effective in the treatment of neck pain and headaches. Avoid massage therapists who are too aggressive. After seeing your massage therapist, you should leave relaxed and not with muscle pain.

After my head injury, I had terrible whiplash. For me, it took seeing several different therapists and using several home neck-care products to control my neck pain, which was triggering my headaches.

Heat and Ice

There are some things you should consider investing in if you have headaches triggered by neck pain. The first thing I recommend is to purchase a high-quality, neck-support pillow. People spend a lot of time in their beds, and during that time it's important to support your neck and back as best as possible. This will promote restful sleep and aid the healing of your neck. You may need to try a couple pillows before you find one that works for you. I have a pillow where the outsides support the top of the head, neck, and jaw with a hollowed-out core in the middle to relieve pressure off my ear and maintain the alignment of my neck. I love this pillow and still use it today.

Second, I recommend investing in heating pads and high-quality ice packs. Heat on your neck encourages muscle relaxation, promotes healing, and improves blood circulation in torn and strained ligaments and muscles. When purchasing a heating pad, make sure it has an automatic shutoff option just in case you fall asleep with it on. You don't want to wake up to a fire in your bed.

A lot of my patients don't like using ice packs on their injuries, but ice is important. Ice decreases inflammation in the muscles and joints and controls pain. Muscles and joints cannot heal if there's ongoing inflammation and swelling in the injury sites. I used ice on my neck several times a day early into my recovery. Large ice packs also helped take the edge off my headaches when my head felt as if it were trapped inside my torturer's vice.

For both heat and ice, it's generally recommended to apply for 20 minutes, with breaks in between applications lasting for at least 20 minutes. Check with your general practitioner or PT to see what they recommend for you.

TAKING MEDICATION

You're probably going to scream, "No, I don't want to have to take a pill every day." I hear this a lot from my patients when I recommend medication. I can reassure you that I have never had a patient squeal with excitement about getting to take a new medication. Nevertheless, preventive medication is necessary to control your headache pain and to prevent you from developing rebound headaches.

There are numerous medications that are used as headache prevention medications. You and your doctor will need to select the best medication that works for you—one that has the least amount of side effects. This process for prescribing medication can be frustrating because it may take a while to figure out which medication will work for you.

The other key component of preventive medications is that they must be slowly increased over time to their recommended therapeutic level. These medications also require that you take them at the recommended therapeutic level for a minimum of two months to see their full effectiveness. This process may take time and patience.

The role of preventive medications is not to eliminate your headaches but to decrease the frequency and intensity of your headaches, limiting the need to use abortive headache medications.

The other important piece to managing headache pain is living a healthy lifestyle. This includes getting high-quality sleep, eating brain-healthy foods, exercise, and stress management. Regardless of medication or therapy, if you don't follow a healthy lifestyle, it will be difficult to control your headaches. Later in this book, I will discuss the healthy lifestyle that I follow and recommend to my patients.

SEEING YOUR GENERAL PRACTITIONER

If the nature of your headaches changes, worsens, or persists, you should see your general practitioner to have your headaches evaluated. A general practitioner can help you identify the type of headache you're suffering from and provide treatment. The treatment for your headaches may include a daily headache preventive medication as well as medications to stop especially painful headaches.

Usually, your health care provider will recommend a daily headache prevention medication if your headaches are frequent and if you need to take over-the-counter medications more than two to three days a week. Because of this, it's best to keep a headache journal. In your headache journal, track the days you have a headache. Keep notes on how intense the headache was, how you treated it, and what may have triggered the headache. This journal will help your general practitioner decide which treatment is best for you and evaluate if your treatment plan is working. I found it helpful to keep track of my headaches in my monthly calendar.

With one or more of these therapies, you may get your head freed from the grips of your maniacal headache torturer. When you have less headache pain, your limited brain energy will be protected, allowing you to use it for work or school while waiting for your brain to heal.

Chapter 8

Fatigue A Constant, Cruel Companion

Following a head injury, you may feel trapped by fatigue. You may feel like Sisyphus pushing his boulder up the mountain every day only to see it roll back down. No matter how much sleep and rest you get, you're still plagued with the daily fatigue that you slowly push up your mountain. At the end of your day, the boulder inevitably rolls over you, leaving you exhausted and unwilling to do it again the next day.

If you complain you're tired, good-intentioned people will tell you to take a nap or go to bed earlier. Most people don't understand how life-altering and relentless brain injury fatigue can be. In their research article "Fatigue After Acquired Brain Injury and Its Impact on Socio-Professional Reintegration," A. Guggisberg, L. Ghauvigné, and J. Pignat said that pathological fatigue is different from normal fatigue and appears more quickly and during nondemanding tasks and that recovery is not complete despite rest.[20] These researchers noted that this fatigue impeded

---

[20] A. Guggisberg, L. Ghauvigné, and J. Pignat, "Fatigue after Acquired Brain Injury and Its Impact on Socio-Professional Reintegration," *Revue Medicalé Suisse* 16, no. 692 (May 2020): 901.

head injury patients from participating in recommended recovery therapies and their ability to return to work. You're too tired, in medical terms, to get better.

INDESCRIBABLE FATIGUE

Dr. Jennie Ponsford and colleagues explain, "More than 60% of patients with traumatic brain injury (TBI) report experiencing fatigue, which interferes with their rehabilitation and daily lifestyle" in their article "Fatigue and Sleep Disturbance Following Traumatic Brain Injury—Their Nature, Causes, and Potential Treatments."[21] This fatigue can be pervasive and affect your cognitive, emotional, and physical energy.

However, researchers still know very little about the relationship between fatigue and brain injury even though it's the most common and lingering symptom. Mary Lou Acimovic and Dr. Gail Denton, in their books, explain that fatigue is related to energy allocation. Before your brain injury, you had 50% of your energy figuratively split equally between cognitive, physical, and emotional functions of the brain, with the other 50% set aside in your cognitive energy reserve.[22]

After an injury, the brain must use all its energy to heal along with other injuries you have sustained, thereby creating a new energy allocation system. After your injury, Mary Lou Acimovic describes that 75% or more of your brain energy is now split between cognitive, physical, and emotional brain functions, leaving between zero and 25% in your energy reserve tank.[23] Let's think about that for a minute. Zero percent on some days! No wonder we're tired.

---

[21] Jennie L. Ponsford et al., "Fatigue and Sleep Disturbance Following Traumatic Brain Injury—Their Nature, Causes, and Potential Treatments," *Journal of Head Trauma Rehabilitation* 27, no. 3 (May–June 2012): 224.

[22] Mary Lou Acimovic, *Mild Traumatic Brain Injury: The Guidebook* (self-published, 2010). Pg 89; Gail L. Denton, *Brainlash: Maximize Your Recovery from Mild Brain Injury* (New York: Demos Health, 2008), 136.

[23] Mary Lou Acimovic, *Mild Traumatic Brain Injury*, 89; Gail L. Denton, *Brainlash*, 136.

Once you've used up your brain energy, there's no additional reserve to tap into. You're done for the day. You are Sisyphus, standing on top of the mountain, watching your boulder roll down, unable to stop it. If you demand more from your brain, it will shut you down and put you to sleep, even if you are driving.

Researchers are also discovering that the brain likes to run efficiently. Research fellow at the Danish Research Centre for Magnetic Resonance Anouk Marsman and colleagues wrote that "the brain works to minimize the resources allocated toward higher cognitive function."[24] In their research, they found the brain performs better when it works efficiently.

After a head injury, areas in your brain processing systems have been disrupted, and brain cell connections have been damaged or severed. In turn, your brain burns a lot more energy inefficiently on simple tasks. Your brain no longer works efficiently. Therefore, you may feel exhausted after just taking a shower because of the energy it took for your brain to work you through the shower.

YOU SLEEP TOO MUCH

You may hear from your doctor that you're tired because you sleep too much. This is not the case for people who have survived a head injury. You have to sleep as much as your brain needs, because while you're sleeping your brain is healing.

Others may recommend you exercise more. This is true for people with healthy brains, but not so for someone healing from a head injury. Exercise is healthy for the brain—just keep in mind that exercise will exact a toll on your brain's energy.

After my car accident, my days consisted of going to work, taking a

---

24 Anouk Marsman et al., "Intelligence and Brain Efficiency: Investigating the Association between Working Memory Performance, Glutamate, and GABA," *Frontiers in Psychiatry* 8 (September 2017): 154, https://www.doi.org/10.3389/fpsyt.2017.00154.

nap in my car at lunch, and working until 5:30 p.m. I would then go home and take a two-hour nap, get up for an hour to get ready for the next day, and go back to sleep until my alarm clock woke me to start the cycle again. My weekends were spent sleeping 12 to 14 hours at night with a two-hour nap midday. I had no social life, and I missed a lot of family time. I was exhausted all the time, crushed by fatigue boulders. Just call me Sisyphus.

I love to be active, whether it's taking a karate class or going on an eight-mile hike. However, when I decide to be active, I also know I will have to pay for it with a nap and extra sleep at night if I want to go back to work on Monday. For me, I can no longer be highly active and work a 40-hour work week. I will talk more about exercise later in this book.

It's important to note that you should not listen to people who minimize your fatigue and say, "Just fake it until you make it." These people do not get your struggle with fatigue. This fatigue is serious. Attempting to push through it or insisting on overdoing it will only put you at risk for physical injury.

There was a time I remember running stairs for exercise. I could feel I was starting to get tired, but I said to myself, "You've got to push through the fatigue to get results." Well, I ignored my brain and continued to leap up the last few stairs. As I told my feet to jump, my brain said, "Ah, no." My feet did not move forward or clear the next step and sent the rest of me flying, causing me to face-plant into the stairs. This was another of my brain's lessons: I was not in charge of my recovery. My brain was the boss of me.

SYMPTOMS

Neuro-fatigue symptoms can be broken down into three categories: physical symptoms, cognitive symptoms, and emotional symptoms. The intensity is different for everyone, but there are some generalities.

Physically you feel as if you move at the speed of a sloth. Emotionally, you may feel like a teenager, wanting to give the middle finger to anyone who irritates you. Cognitively, you may not even be able to decide what you want for dinner.

Physical fatigue symptoms may include the following:

- Waking up feeling tired
- Feeling tired all the time, day after day
- Feeling fatigued after minimal activity
- Taking longer to get things done
- Feeling a relentless need to lie down and go to sleep
- Worsening of headaches, dizziness, pain, or other head injury symptoms
- Decreasing coordination or balance

Cognitive fatigue may include these symptoms:

- An inability to decide, plan, or organize
- Brain fog or slow thinking
- No motivation
- Confusion
- Difficulty maintaining focus
- An inability to absorb information or directions

Emotional fatigue often includes the symptoms below:

- Irritability or grumpiness
- Becoming easily frustrated
- Frequent mood swings
- Feelings of sadness, anxiety, or depression
- Difficulty controlling your temper

Living with Head Injury Fatigue

Knowing your limits and protecting your brain energy are strategies to employ when recovering from a head injury. You need to learn when to take breaks *before* you become exhausted and unable to function. Once you have this skill down, you can pace yourself throughout the day, interlacing moments of work with periods of rest.

Remember, pacing is a hard skill to learn. Many people without brain injuries have a hard time pacing themselves too, so be patient with yourself.

Another strategy is creating a quiet and restful home. Dim bright lights, limit unnecessary sounds (how many of us leave the TV on?), and clear out any visual clutter, such as piles of laundry on the couch or paperwork stacked up on the dining room table. Allow your brain to enjoy the calm quiet of your home.

You may ask, "What if I live with children?" If you have small children, you'll need to employ noise-canceling earbuds or headphones when your children's happy, gleeful squeals and giggles become too overwhelming. You will still hear and monitor your little ones, but give your brain a rest by filtering out loud noises.

I live with a pre-teen and a teenager. I've asked them to wear headphones when they're using their smart devices, to turn off the volume of video games, and to have their phone conversations in their room or outside. We also don't have the TV on unless someone is sitting and watching it. Since our home is normally quiet, we also tend to speak in normal to low voices.

As with having a home clear of clutter while sharing it with children, all I can say is good luck. For me this is mission impossible because my kids are slobs. So, I had to let go of the expectation of a 100% clean and organized home. Maybe when the kids move out? Instead, I created spaces within my home that my family knew were Mom's spots. These spaces I can keep clutter-free and escape to when the house is overwhelming me.

Eating healthy and getting quality sleep, exercise, and plenty of outside time will also help promote your brain's healing and protect or even add to its energy banks.

SEE A SPECIALIST

I remember being perplexed by my neurologist's recommendation that I see an endocrinologist. Endocrinologists help people with hormone imbalances related to their glands. They diagnose and treat diseases such as diabetes and thyroid disorders. What does that have to do with the brain?

I was surprised to learn that researchers have been studying pituitary dysfunction caused by a TBI. The pituitary is a pea-sized gland in the brain that can be damaged from a head injury. These researchers found that TBI is one of the top reasons for decreased hormone production by the pituitary gland.[25] Decreased hormone production by the pituitary gland can cause symptoms such as fatigue, headaches, and dizziness. Ah ha!

The endocrinologist can screen you for hormonal deficiencies by examining your MRI, reviewing your blood tests, and using procedures that induce and measure hormonal response to stress. Two of the most common diagnoses are hypopituitarism and growth hormone deficiency.

Hypopituitarism is when your pituitary gland doesn't make enough hormones to tell your other glands in your body to get to work—meaning your body is a soldier left without a drill sergeant. Growth hormone deficiency can cause you to gain weight at your waistline or make you feel depressed, anxious, or fatigued.

Züleyha Karaca and colleagues, in their article "GH and Pituitary Hormone Alterations after Traumatic Brain Injury," found that patients with TBI–induced growth hormone deficiency had difficulty with cognitive abilities and mood control.[26] When hormonal deficiencies were treated, patients reported improvement in their quality of life.

I ended up seeing three endocrinologists. The first endocrinologist was within my health plan, and this doctor disagreed with my behavioral

---

25 Züleyha Karaca et al., "GH and Pituitary Hormone Alterations after Traumatic Brain Injury," *Progress in Molecular Biology and Translational Science* 138 (2016): 167–191, https://www.doi.org/10.1016/bs.pmbts.2015.10.010.
26 Karaca et al., "GH and Pituitary Hormone Alterations," 167-191.

neurologist and recommended that I exercise more and sleep less. It was obvious to me that this endocrinologist was not knowledgeable about head injuries.

I saw another endocrinologist who told me to stop taking my birth control pills. Since I sat in his office for two hours waiting to see him, I was able to see he told all his female patients the same thing.

The third doctor was the charm. This endocrinologist specialized in head injuries. After a blood test, a comprehensive exam, and a glucagon stimulation test, my doctor explained to me that I had borderline neuroendocrine dysfunction with growth hormone insufficiency. He believed that this was the cause of my unrelenting fatigue.

Receiving this diagnosis meant a lot to me. It reassured me that I was not a lazy ass and that there were multiple reasons for my fatigue. I also discovered that I didn't need to exercise more, sleep less, or stop taking my birth control pills.

The above is an example of why I tell my patients to advocate for themselves. Here are ways to do that:

- Find a provider whom you trust.
- Take a supportive friend or family member to all your health appointments.
- Do your own research.
- Don't be afraid to seek a second or even a third opinion.
- You may need to consider paying out of pocket to see a specialist not covered by your health insurance. That can be expensive, but the cost of seeing an outside provider is like making an investment in the success of your future.

Fatigue can be caused by multiple medical conditions, some of which can be treated. Therefore, it's important to follow up with your health care provider and let them know of your fatigue so other health conditions can be ruled out.

Chapter 9

Your Inner Hulk Behavior Changes after a Head Injury

Everyone has an inner Hulk that lives inside their brain, but most of us are pretty good at keeping him under control. Head injuries make it more difficult. Sometimes we may let him slip out, making us more emotional, irritable, sad, angry, or anxious. Something, especially stress, may trigger us, and we suddenly snap. We may lose control of our ability to reason. We may start yelling, hitting the wall, or throwing things across the room.

Following a head injury, you may feel less inhibited and more prone to letting your emotions get the best of you. You may behave in inappropriate ways and disregard the consequences of your actions. You may even be self-aware, but you will constantly feel the struggle to keep these symptoms under control. As smart as Bruce Banner is, even he has difficulty controlling the big green monster lurking inside him.

BAD BEHAVIOR AND DECISIONS

After a head injury, it's common for the areas in your brain responsible for processing good judgment, reasoning, and self-awareness to be damaged. Poor brain function in these critical "adulting" skills will be reflected in your behavior.

Your self-monitoring and good-judgment brain functions help you weigh the consequences of your behavior, actions, and decision-making. Self-monitoring helps you judge socially appropriate behavior and allows you to understand the limits of your capabilities. If your self-monitoring, judgment, and reasoning skills were disrupted during your head injury, say hello to the Hulk. Until these brain processes heal, I strongly recommend that you seek help from a trusted family member or friend to help you recognize when your inner Hulk is beginning to take over your brain and behavior. These loved ones can help you move away from or avoid situations that trigger your inner Hulk and remind you to use your therapy strategies to help you regain control.

My inner Hulk was awful. She would snap at people, interrupt others while they were talking, and replace my adjectives with cuss words. I would say things out loud that I normally would not let escape my lips, and I remember not caring how those words affected others. My post–head injury behavior ended up affecting my personal relationships and my credibility at work.

When my self-awareness returned, I was able to look back on my behavior and see things I wished I had not done. By noting my mistakes and identifying what triggered my behavior, I was able to avoid repeating the bad behavior. I also started to communicate better with my family, and when I started to feel irritable or overwhelmed, they knew not to take my grumpiness personally.

At work when I started to feel stress or overwhelmed, I applied strategies such as taking deep breaths or walking away from the stressful situation. When I was stuck in a meeting I could not escape from, I learned to keep my mouth shut and remind myself to do more listening instead of talking. Over time I was able to earn my credibility back with my colleagues.

I remember the moment my self-awareness returned. I was hanging clothes up in my closet and thinking about previous conversations I'd had with my friends when a strange sensation caused a sinking feeling in my chest. I stopped midway while hanging up a shirt, sat down, and analyzed this strange feeling. I started to feel sorry for the words I'd said. I realized the sensation was remorse and regret—feelings that I'd not felt for the past three months. I was not aware that these brain processes had stopped working for me.

Despite feeling regretful and embarrassed for my past behavior, I was also happy and excited. This was a good sign that my brain was healing. If my self-monitoring and awareness returned, this gave me hope that my other brain functions would return in time too.

Fortunately, for most people these areas of the brain start to come back online early in recovery. Until then, put your feelings, thoughts, and emotions down in a journal so that you can learn what's going on in your head. Also look to family and friends for guidance with understanding and controlling your inner Hulk.

PERSONALITY CHANGES

After your head injury, you may look into a mirror and see the same person you were before your head injury. However, inside you may feel you're not that same person anymore.

Following my accident I felt as if my body had survived but the person I'd been had died. The things I pursued and enjoyed no longer interested me. I felt I couldn't trust my perception of the world or the people around me. I also lost the ability to understand humor. For a while, I felt lost inside my head.

You may also feel that your personality has changed. Though you may have been outgoing before your head injury, it's possible you now find that you prefer staying home with a warm cup of coffee while sitting and watching birds fly in and out of the trees in your yard. Before your head injury, you may have been quiet and reserved. Now you might find yourself speaking up at work or in class and are more willing to take on outgoing challenges. You may have considered yourself more of a left-brain person who liked organizing and planning, and you now find yourself reveling for hours in paints, clay, music, or poetry.

Before my head injury, I was a basic T-shirt–and–jeans gal who did not have time for cooking or organizing my home because I was off to my next adventure of traveling or seeing friends. After my injury, I turned into a fashion queen who loved to shop, accessorize my outfits, and wear red lipstick. I preferred to stay home to clean, organize, garden, cook, and complete home-improvement projects. So weird, right?

Some of my personality changes were good. For instance, I was a more easygoing person who enjoyed relaxing at home. However, it came with a price. My family saw a dramatic drop in our social life. We lost touch with some of our friends. My kids missed out on playdates and time hanging out with their friends. We stopped going out to dinner or seeing a movie for family night. We even stopped traveling.

As a family we stopped training at the dojo, and this meant our kids lost an avenue they used to find and make new friends. As time passed, we became more and more isolated within our own family bubble. This was hard on my kids.

Three months after my head injury, my husband had to quit his job as a martial arts instructor so that he could support me as I strived to continue working in order to keep a roof over our heads and food on the table. My husband was forced to assume all the household chores. He essentially became a single parent to our children because I could not stay awake after working a full day. This was hard for him because he lost his self-identity, was socially isolated from friends, and came under a lot of stress from taking care of me and our children. Later on down the road, my husband ended up needing to be treated for generalized anxiety disorder.

If you notice changes in your personality, pay attention to them. These changes can be good, but they can also affect your loved ones. The changes may lead to a new lifestyle for you and your family, and they can change your family's core values. If needed, solicit the insights of your trusted family, friends, or family counselor to help identify and cope with these new changes.

Monitor for Risk of Suicide

During your recovery it's reasonable to be sad, frustrated, or angry, but if you find that you constantly feel helpless or worthless, lose interest in doing things you enjoyed in the past, have difficulty with sleep, or notice a change in your appetite, you may have depression. If you have thoughts of death or if you're considering hurting yourself, your depression needs to be medically evaluated and treated.

At times during my recovery, I had thoughts that my family would be better off without me. I felt worthless and thought nothing I did was good enough. Occasionally I displayed impulsive, risky behavior that, frankly, put my life in danger.

Episodes of road rage happened a few times. I'd scream like a banshee as I slammed my foot on the gas and sped dangerously down the road, often taking tight turns at high speeds, not caring if I crashed and died. Fortunately, these episodes were brief.

Even though I never admitted having these episodes or thoughts to my neuropsychologist, the results of my neurocognitive testing showed that I tended to downplay my health concerns and was at risk of burning out under the stress of working and trying to recover. Fortunately, with medication, talking to a psychologist who specialized in head injuries, and time, those thoughts faded away.

Some people need to go through a grieving process after a head injury. This grieving process can be challenging and complex. You may have problems with emotional behavioral issues, as I did, which can put you at risk for hurting yourself. If this is true for you, find help from a mental health specialist who specializes in head injuries. Don't suffer through these symptoms alone. Get the help you need, because you and your brain are worth it.

SYMPTOMS

Below are the common behavioral symptoms after a head injury. It may be necessary to do a checklist of the ones that apply to you so you can inform a health care provider and find necessary treatment.

- Irritability
- Bursts of anger
- Mood swings
- Anxiety or fearfulness
- Exaggerated startle response
- Easily frustrated
- Apathy, low motivation, lack of self-limitation
- Easily overwhelmed or overstimulated
- Symptoms of depression
- Hopelessness
- Sadness (mild to overwhelming)
- Guilt
- Grief
- Loss of sense of self
- Change in personality
- Impulsiveness or loss of inhibition
- Lack of self-awareness
- Poor judgment
- Post-traumatic stress or post-injury psychological reactions
- Nightmares

SEE A SPECIALIST

Would you expect someone to "think more positive" to fix their diabetes? No, you would expect they would get treated by a specialist. Mental health is a medical condition that warrants the same kind of care.

When you seek a specialist, make sure they have experience and training in caring for patients with head injuries. Some of these specialists are psychiatrists, neuropsychologists, and family counselors.

While practicing as a neuro–nurse practitioner, I've found that some of my patients misunderstand the difference between a neurologist and a psychiatrist. When I recommend my patients to see a psychiatrist, they often ask why. A psychiatrist is a medical doctor who can determine if you have a mental health problem that may have been brought on or worsened by your head injury. They can also prescribe medications to treat various mental health disorders and behavior issues. A psychiatrist can also help treat sleep disorders.

A neuropsychologist can help you learn how to rein in your inner Hulk, screen you for additional compounding mental health conditions, and identify post-traumatic stress disorder. A neuropsychologist will teach you coping strategies that will help you cope with daily challenges. They can also test and measure your intellectual, cognitive, and vocational skills and identify your personality characteristics.

I saw a neuropsychologist and learned a great deal about my brain after my head injury. I was reassured that I was not a big, crazy jerk and that my inner emotional turmoil was a result of my head injury affecting my concentration and attention. This explained my irritability and frustration when someone or something disrupted my focus.

A head injury does not only affect the person who is injured. Its impact ripples into the person's family life, work, and circle of friends. When your behavior starts to cause conflict within your family, consider acquiring the help of a family counselor. You can also think about participating in a support group for head injury survivors and their caregivers. I will talk more about family role changes later in this book.

Changes in your personality and behavior after a head injury are one of the hardest symptoms to overcome when healing from a head injury. For most people, these symptoms resolve early in their recovery. For me the changes in my personality were permanent. If your personality and behavior changes persist, don't suffer alone. Seek the help you, your family, and your brain need.

Section III

Tools and Strategies

Chapter 10
My Tool Bag

IT CAN BE GRUELING when the world keeps spinning even though your life has been turned upside down. Despite the fact that you've sustained a head injury, your responsibilities will pile up like a dark, daunting mountain. Your boss or instructors will be calling, emailing, and texting you, wanting to know when you will return to work even though all you want to do is take a nap.

I returned to work unprepared, not knowing my brain needed support to get through the day's demands. But after reading books, searching the internet, and seeking advice from specialists, with some trial and error, I was eventually able to assemble a bag of tools and strategies to help me continue to work while my brain healed.

In this section, we'll talk about the tools I use to get through a day at work while recovering from my brain injury.

INSIDE MY TOOL BAG

- **Journaling:** Journaling is a powerful tool that will aid you in identifying your symptoms and tracking the progress of your healing. A recovery journal will also be a haven where you can reflect on the swirling thoughts and emotions that come with the frustration of a head injury.

- **Give yourself a break:** Being motivated, managing your time, and getting organized are higher brain functions that need a lot of energy to power. This is energy your brain is not able to provide while it's healing.

- **Light and sound sensitivity:** After a head injury, you may cringe under lights and wonder why the world is too loud. You may also have the attention span of a gnat, making it difficult for you to focus while at work and school.

- **Brain breaks:** While your brain is healing, it's important to take frequent breaks. I'll talk more about how to do this later in this book.

- **Get off on the right foot:** You may find that getting ready and arriving on time to planned appointments is difficult after a head injury. The last thing you want is to use up all your brain energy just to get out the door. You'll need to plan and start getting ready earlier, perhaps even the night before.

- **Managing a to-do list:** After a head injury, you may find you need to keep a list to help you remember the things you need to get done.

- **New ways of learning:** Learning is a complex brain function that can get knocked off-line after a head injury. But you *have not* lost the ability to learn. So, take a deep, calming breath and read about new ways you and your brain may prefer to learn while you're recovering from a head injury.

These tools and strategies have been a lifesaver for me and supported my return to work after my head injury. Hopefully these tools and strategies will help you avoid making the same mistakes I made and smooth your return to work or school.

Chapter 11

Journaling
Yes, You're Making Progress:
It's Right There in Writing

BRAIN INJURIES REQUIRE PATIENCE. It's often very hard to see your progress because recovery is incremental. It may take days, weeks, or even months before you start getting back to the person who resembles your normal self. So, imagine how nice it would be to have someone who could look at you every day and say, "I see improvement. You're definitely getting better." This person is you, via a journal.

A recovery journal might be the most powerful tool you will use in solving the mysteries of your head injury. Dr. Gail Denton says that "journaling helps you notice and remember how far you have come."[27] By writing down your symptoms every day and being aware of what's going on inside your head, you'll be able to see the incremental steps you're taking in your recovery. I recommend journaling in a notebook.

---

[27] Gail L. Denton, *Brainlash: Maximize Your Recovery from Mild Brain Injury* (New York: Demos Health, 2008), 202.

Once you write out your symptoms, your observations will aid you in flagging aggravating influencers that cause your symptoms, which are known as triggers. Recognizing what triggers your symptoms will help you implement strategies and tools to support your efforts while your brain heals. Triggers, as I've said earlier, can be noise, bright light, or emotional stress.

One month after my car accident, I started a journal. When I started, it was just a place for me to vent my frustrations. The journaling eventually helped me see that, four months after my car accident, my symptoms were getting worse and not better.

I wrote, "I am now determined to get the care I deserve and desperately need for my concussion." I was tired of trying to get better on my own.

It wasn't until 2019 that I started to understand a pattern with my episodes of regression and their triggers. It took me over four years of journaling and self-reflection on my recovery to piece together the triggers that sidelined my recovery efforts and drained my cognitive energy. I'm hoping this chapter will help you figure out your triggers a lot sooner.

The first component is to find the triggers that drain your battery. This is where journaling comes into play. Every day you should write in your journal about how things during the day affected you, the impact they made on your head injury symptoms, and your recovery.

Take the Pain from the Brain and Put It on the Page

Journaling has many other benefits as well. It can support mindfulness, decrease worry and anxiety, and aid in managing emotions and stress.[28] During your recovery it's best to look back at your progress and accomplishments. The last thing you want to do is to get stuck focusing on what

---

[28] "Mental Health Benefits of Journaling," WebMD, October 25, 2021, https://www. webmd.com/mental-health/mental-health-benefits-of-journaling.

you're not able to do today or to waste energy on worrying about the future.

Most people see the most improvements in their symptoms the first two years of their recovery. After this time your healing accomplishments will become subtle and less frequent. Your journal will help you track these small improvements, help stave off doubtful thoughts, and calm frustrations as you patiently wait for your brain to heal. This is when your journal becomes your supportive friend.

The first-year anniversary after my car crash, I reflected on the previous year of journaling. Because of my journal, I was able to see that my neck injury had finally healed. I had less drowsiness with driving, fewer days of brain fog, and the ability to stay awake after work a few nights a week. I also wrote that work stress often derailed my efforts to heal and that I was going to need more time to recover.

There's something cathartic about writing down your thoughts, emotions, and ideas on a piece of paper. For people with a TBI, it can also help you observe and track the inner workings—all your moods and thoughts—of your brain. I think of it as a verbal or linguistic electroencephalogram.

My journal reminded me that the first few weeks after my car accident, I couldn't make coffee and toast at the same time. I had such a hard time multitasking other simple tasks that I used to be able to do on autopilot. It was nice to see how far I had come from that time.

This is why journaling is important in the early phases of your recovery. Journaling places your thoughts out of your head and onto paper. This transference of ideas, worries, and to-do lists will reduce the drain on your cognitive energy, decrease your mental load, and take some stress off your brain. Once your worries and fretful thoughts are on paper, you can get a clearer perspective of what's going on in your head. This perspective will help you work through and manage your mood, negative thoughts, emotions, and behavior issues, allowing you to strengthen your emotional control while around others.

For some, a brain injury might shut off your filter—the mechanism in your brain that tells you what is and isn't appropriate to say or do in certain situations. Journaling will help prevent you from saying things to others in frustration or anger that you will regret later.

After you completed your own reflections, you can decide to share your struggles with a trusted friend or family member. If not, it's still a great space for you to do a quick self-check. Getting down all your rampant thoughts and developing an understanding of situations will inevitably make you feel less anxious, uncomfortable, irritable, or angry.

Your journaling will assist you in analyzing the effectiveness of coping strategies, therapies, treatments, counseling, support groups, and medication. It's the foundation for all the work that will be necessary in your recovery.

The other nice thing about journaling is that it doesn't talk back. Your journal will not talk over you, interrupt you, or make you lose your train of thought. You also won't have to apologize to it. No matter what you say to it or how many cuss words you write in it, your journal will always lend an ear.

Journaling Your Symptoms

Telling a specialist that you have dizziness is not helpful. But saying you have noticed a sense of dizziness while working on a large-screen computer when you're moving your eyes to various spots on the screen and scrolling up or down is another story. You've now handed your health care provider detailed information to help them in their assessment of your complaint of dizziness. You and your provider now know that you have dizziness from visual tracking and that you would benefit from neuro–physical therapy.

What if you said working on the computer for longer than 20 minutes gives you a headache? You have identified that your trigger to your post-concussion headaches is working on the computer without an eye break. You now know that your headache is your brain telling you that it needs a moment to rest before moving forward.

In my practice, people don't remember these details when they see a specialist unless they have the details written down in front of them. I see patients forget questions they want to ask, and they also forget what was discussed at the visit. Keeping a recovery journal will help to keep all your care information in one spot. Your journal becomes your memory storage, remembering things your brain cannot remember on its own for now.

Your journaling does not need to be complicated. I recommend using a spiral notebook with storage pockets. These pockets can hold receipts, therapy exercise handouts, and printed medical information. Use your journal to keep all your important information during your recovery in one organized place.

If you need some help getting started, here's how I like to make entries:

- Start your journal entries with the date of your injury.
- Journal your visits with your recovery providers, financial advisers, and legal appointments.
- Write down your accomplishments and any improvements in your functioning.
- List all the symptoms you've noticed since your injury.
- Go back and review the list of symptoms that are in this book.
- Add any additional symptoms that you have.
- Recheck the symptoms list and list your own symptoms every three months for the first six months and then every six months after.
- Check off the symptoms that have resolved after six months and add any new symptoms you need to start monitoring.
- Journal important information you want to share with your provider along with any questions you'd like to ask at your next visit.

You should take this journal everywhere you go. At the beginning of the day, carry it with you. At the end of the day, place it by your bed.

Later in your recovery, use your journal to keep track of bills, a to-do list, and financial goals, such as a budget and a list of all your expenses.

KEEPING A JOURNAL AT WORK

I believe my journals kept me from hurting my relationship with my husband and destroying my relationships with my children, friends, and colleagues. My journal helped me keep a lot of crazy, off-the-rails thoughts and frustrations to myself. It also replaced my brain filter and has continued to help me bite my tongue when I get emotionally charged, and it was a big reason I was able to keep my job.

I know after my traumatic brain injury I struggled with various issues such as paranoia, insecurities, and increased sensitivity. I felt as if people were out to get me and things hurt my feelings more easily. The journal helped me process those feelings and thoughts. It gave me time to step back and see the whole picture and what triggered me.

If you're able to work, I recommend keeping a separate work journal. In this journal you can track your progress, efficiency, setbacks, frustrations, distractions, and difficulty with time management. Then when you go back and read those recorded workday challenges, it will help you to establish a few coping mechanisms to mitigate those identified workplace challenges and their effects on your performance.

In your work journal, you should write down important work conversations and meetings. For my work journal, I even printed important emails and stapled them into my work journal. This helped me keep track of timelines and important information I needed to reference later.

As you keep your work journal, you will be able to look back on the days, weeks, and months of your work and identify areas in which you need to develop strategies or utilize tools that will support your overall work performance.

Having a work and personal journal will allow you to see your healing progress over time. Although you might often be frustrated or even sad, pulling out your journal can help to remind yourself of how far you have come along during your recovery.

Chapter 12

Tools for Work and School
Light and Sound

A FEW MONTHS INTO my brain injury and subsequent recovery, I decided to go back to work—not a good idea. I remember on my first day it felt as if everyone I met was talking too loud or too fast. The smallest office noise sounded like firecrackers. Even something like the hum of a refrigerator sounded loud. The clicking sound of someone typing on their keyboard made me want to slap that person over the head with said keyboard.

If you don't know what light and sound sensitivity is, well, it's like the beginning of a superhero movie when the superhero is just getting their powers and is hypersensitive to everything around them. They can hear the mice crawling down in the sewers, a bird's wingbeats, and the neighbor coughing three doors down. The only difference is that your superpower is at times downright debilitating.

PLEASE, DON'T SHINE THE LIGHT ON ME

In movies, we know the superheroes need to protect themselves when they're first learning about and developing their powers. Likewise, you need to protect your brain.

After a head injury, your brain will be happiest in a dark, quiet room. When you grow stronger, you'll need to return to the brightly lit world that people have grown accustomed to living in.

Light sensitivity is commonly reported by people after a brain injury. Your light sensitivity could stem from several issues. One common reason is that your brain doesn't have the energy to filter the light entering the brain from your eyes. Other causes of light sensitivity can be due to visual changes after a head injury.

I made the mistake of returning to work immediately after a brain injury. I was highly susceptible to sound and light, and it was only over the course of a couple years, a lot of research, and meeting with several specialists that I came to develop my own strategies and tools to help protect my brain's sensory input from the daily bombardment of an overstimulating work environment. I have collected those strategies and tools below.

FLUORESCENT LIGHTS SUCK

Fluorescent lights are hard on the brain because the light is not constant light. Fluorescent lights flicker and are known to cause eye strain, eye disease, headaches, disrupted sleep patterns, and decreased focus in people with healthy brains. Dr. Helen Walls, Kelvin Walls, and Geza Benke reported in their article "Eye Disease Resulting from Increased Use of Fluorescent Lighting as a Climate Change Mitigation Strategy" that fluorescent light increases development of cataracts.[29]

Fluorescent lights drain your brain's energy, worsen brain injury

---

[29] Helen Walls, Kelvin Walls, and Geza Benke, "Eye Disease Resulting from Increased Use of Fluorescent Lighting as a Climate Change Mitigation Strategy," *American Journal of Public Health* 101, no. 12 (December 2011): 2222–25, https://www.doi.org/10.2105/AJPH.2011.300246.

symptoms, and decrease your brain's cognitive functioning. But don't feel bad—it happens to "regular people" as well. Sadly, businesses and schools use fluorescent lights as a cost-saving means of lighting their buildings.

Meik Wiking, author of *The Little Book of Hygge: Danish Secrets to Happy Living,* provides this perspective on fluorescent lights: "the closest you will ever come to seeing vampires burned by daylight is by inviting a group of Danes for a hygge dinner and then placing them under a fluorescent light … they will squint, trying to examine the torture device you have placed in the ceiling."[30]

To promote the highest performance of your brain, work under natural light. However, that may not be an option if you work in a windowless office. One option is to ask your employer to switch out the fluorescent light over your workspace to a warmer incandescent light or install a dimmer to dim the harsh glare of the light.

If your employer is unwilling to make changes to the fluorescent lights, block the lights' harmful effects on your brain with other tools, such as wearing dark glasses or blue-light–filtering glasses. These can be found on the internet and can be worn over your regular eyeglasses. You can also wear a light-blocking hat with your glasses.

Some other options are fluorescent-filtering light covers and blockers that can be attached to the walls of your cubical. An adjustable clamp umbrella or two can also be installed onto your desk to block light glaring on to you and your computer.

HOME LIGHTING

Don't forget the lights in your home, as dimming will protect your brain's healing. Consider switching out fluorescent lights for incandescent lightbulbs. Lightbulbs that give off warm gold, glowing light are also better than

---

[30] Meik Wiking, *The Little Book of Hygge: Danish Secrets to Happy Living,* (New York: William Morrow, 2017), 6.

the glare of pure-white lightbulbs. You can also switch out high-wattage bulbs for a lower-wattage bulb.

One of my patients who suffered from light sensitivity installed lower-wattage LED lights in all his light fixtures and installed dimmers in all his light switches. Dimming the lights in his home helped decrease the intensity and frequency of his post-concussion headaches. Or you can do what I did: when one of my lightbulbs burned out, I just didn't replace it.

Rest assured, as your brain heals, you will become less sensitive to most lighting in your home. As time passed, I even started to replace my burned-out bulbs in my light fixtures.

BLUE LIGHT

Blue light is a light that is emitted from fluorescent lights but also from many computers and media devices. Richard Inger and colleagues reported in their article "Potential Biological and Ecological Effects of Flickering Artificial Light" that blue lights are known to cause "headaches, visual effects, and both neurological and physiological symptoms."[31] After a head injury, people are more sensitive to the effects of blue light emanating from media devices.

There are several blue-light–filtering tools available that you can choose from to protect your brain's energy. There are blue-light filters that can be placed on computer screens, tablets, and smartphones. As I mentioned before, there are also blue-light–filtering glasses that can be worn over your own prescription glasses. I've also found that my optometrist office offers prescription glasses with blue-light blocking. Maybe your optometrist office does too.

Researchers have found evidence that people with traumatic brain injuries, when provided with light-filtering lenses, saw that "reading rates

---

[31] Richard Inger et al., "Potential Biological and Ecological Effects of Flickering Artificial Light," *PLOS One* 9, no. 5 (May 2014): 2, https://doi.org/10.1371/journal.pone.0098631.

enhanced up to 39% above that measured in the presence of nearpoint optical correction alone."[32]

You should limit your exposure to blue light as much as possible. Blue light is a drain on your brain's energy reserves. Early into your recovery, you should avoid all use of personal media devices and avoid watching TV and scrolling through social media accounts. As you heal you can slowly return to using these devices. Also be sure to turn off your devices the moment a headache, dizziness, or fatigue starts.

It helps to note the amount of time you're able to tolerate your exposure to blue light and stay within that limit until you have more brain energy. As time progresses, you will see your endurance improve.

When you're able to finish a workday without having to come home and take a nap, this is usually a good indicator that you're developing more brain energy. When your brain injury symptoms are well controlled, this is a good sign that you can begin using your personal devices at home.

Other ways to limit exposure to blue light is to not read, analyze, or study information off your computer screen if it can be printed on paper. The other advantage of printing an article or presentation off the computer is that you can take the printed pages and read them in a quiet and darker area, giving your brain a break from filtering out environmental distractions while allowing it to focus on the printed text.

I recommend organizing printed material in a three-ring binder with marked color tabs for easy reference. If you cannot print what is on your computer screen, grab a piece of paper. Take the paper and place its edge along the sentence you are reading. This paper will support your eyes' gaze as it follows the sentence along. This way your brain saves some energy by not having to focus your eyes as much. The paper's edge will guide your gaze and keep it from skipping down a line or two.

---

[32] Mary M. Jackowski et al., "Photophobia in Patients with Traumatic Brain Injury: Uses of Light-Filtering Lenses to Enhance Contrast Sensitivity and Reading Rate," *NeuroRehabilitation* 6, no. 3 (1996): 193, https://www.doi.org/10.3233/NRE-1996-6305.

If you're interested in playing brain games, don't play video games or brain games on your smart devices. This is unnecessary exposure to blue light. Instead, there are brain game books that you can order off the internet or find at local pharmacies.

Computer and Smartphone Tips

Don't forget that dimming the brightness of your computer screen helps reduce eye strain and headaches. This setting is under the Brightness display. Some devices also have the option to limit blue-light exposure. For my iPhone this is under the Night Shift setting. When you activate this setting, your phone will automatically go into Dark Mode at sunset. This setting is much gentler at the end of the day when your eyes are tired.

A lot of computers and smart devices also have accessibility features in their settings. With these features you can change the contrast of your text, enlarge the size of your text, and use a supportive setting, such as Spoken Content.

Large text with increased contrast helps reduce eye strain and makes reading easier for your brain. The Spoken Content setting is a wonderful feature with which you can highlight text and have your device read it out loud for you. Listening to text gives you a chance to look away from your device and rest your eyes. Listening to text as compared to reading consumes less brain energy.

These small, little changes can make a big difference in preserving your brain energy for other tasks and allow you to work longer on complicated tasks, which can help to improve your performance at work and in school.

The World Is Just Too Damn Loud

Four years after my head injury, I was sent to a specialist who diagnosed me with binocular vision dysfunction. Based on a questionnaire I filled out, they also told me that I was sound sensitive. Well, I thought to myself, this explains why everyone's conversation voices seem so loud.

Much to my surprise, the doctor recommended I try noise-canceling headphones, and I was immediately shocked at the difference. When the doctor tested my gait, he told me I walked straighter when I had the headphones on. Sometimes a superhero needs a device to help them control their powers. After a few months with my headphones, I realized I had more energy.

Sound sensitivity can be a persistent symptom after a head injury. It can be annoying and so overwhelming that your brain will just shut down. It's awful. It makes you grumpy and tired, and focusing feels like mission impossible.

Some people don't realize that they have sound sensitivity. You may suffer from a sense of anxiety and irritability when you're out and about in the world. Confusion while out shopping might be commonplace as your decision skills slowly drag to a halt. You may flounder while attempting to focus on a conversation between you and a friend in a restaurant, or you may have difficulty paying attention to someone speaking to you at a seminar with multiple conversations occurring around you. Difficulty comprehending what you're reading if there are people or noises around you might also occur. You may have an increase in fatigue or headaches after hanging out with friends at a party or bar.

One way you may notice that you suffer from sound sensitivity is if you place noise-canceling headphones or earbuds on and feel yourself slip into quiet serenity with a sigh of relief.

Huge, Brightly Colored Headphones

These tools essentially create a sound filter for your brain. While your brain normally filters out these distracting sounds, it doesn't have the energy for this task when it's trying to heal. This is also why sounds seem so much louder to a person with a brain injury as compared to their healthy counterparts.

The options can be as low tech as simply as placing earplugs in your ears whenever you are in a loud environment. Opting for high-tech options like sound-canceling headphones or earbuds that connect to your smartphone and have an app that lets you control the amount of sound in your ears is another solution. Some devices even allow you to control the direction of your earbuds' focus on the sounds around you. These devices allow you to focus the earbuds at a conversation that is occurring across the table or on the TV across the room. I have a pair of these, and I think they are awesome!

If you're as sound sensitive as I am, you can wear two devices at the same time. When I am at work, I wear both my sound-canceling earbuds along with my noise-canceling headphones. Oftentimes, when wearing my noise-canceling device, I will also pipe in music to further counteract people's voices.

The other advantage of wearing headphones at work or school is that it deters people from bothering you while you are working at your computer or laptop. People also don't expect you to participate in idle conversation when you have your headphones on. This helps reduce the times throughout the day when your focus is fractured by others. This is a total win, right?

There are also white noise machines that you can place on your desk to help drown out other distracting noises. If possible, request a desk away from audible distractions such as printers, copiers, ringing telephones at a reception desk, bathrooms, and the breakroom or water cooler where employees tend to gather for conversations.

With these simple interventions you'll be able to focus better and work and study a little bit longer.

ROUND AND ROUND

As you sit focused in front of your work, you may find your eyes and mind leaving your work intermittently. This can be for a second, or it may lead to five minutes of watching a squirrel play in a tree.

This is okay if you're simply trying to read a book in your local park, but it's not okay if you have a paper to write for school or an important email to compose to your boss. These distractions drain your brain's energy. Every time your focus is pulled away by a visual distraction, it's breaking your focus. When your attention is pulled away by a distraction, your brain has to spend energy to ignore the distraction and refocus your attention back to the task you were working on. As the day goes on, these efforts pile up and take a toll on your already limited brain energy.

This is why it's important to block visual distractions when you're working or studying. If possible, request a desk at work or study in an area with few to no people. Choose a desk that faces a wall or a corner. If that's not an option, create barriers to block your peripheral vision from the movement occurring around you. This can be a cubical wall, a desk lamp, a small shelf with books, or even a large plant on your desk.

Stop Scaring the Crap Out of Me

Another common distraction is co-workers disrupting your concentration by walking up to your desk. Even people who have healthy brains sometimes get annoyed by this, but for a person with a brain injury, it's like death by a thousand cuts.

When I'm at work, I'm usually sitting at my computer, facing a corner, wearing dark glasses and headphones. Every time someone comes up to my desk and interrupts my focus, they scare the crap out of me, making me squeak in surprise or say "shit" out loud. I'm glad my co-workers think it's funny.

If you can, request that co-workers send you an email or leave a voice-mail instead of coming to your desk. If the message is more urgent, then request that they send you a text. This type of communication allows you to decide the moment you're ready to transition from your current project to place your focus on their message.

Fortunately, my co-workers kindly send me staff messages, saying that they're coming to my desk prior to their arrival. This helps me anticipate their approach. Some people have also opted to tap lightly on the back of my chair instead of on the shoulder, which has also helped. Maybe your fellow workers can do this for you.

The more you limit and block out these distractions, the longer you will be able to maintain your focus on your work. You'll also be able to save your brain's energy for working or studying a little bit longer and driving home safely.

CONCLUSION

I'm still sensitive to light and sound. While I'm working, I'll see a bird in my periphery and instantly become distracted. No, it's not a useful superpower, and it's not going to help you save anyone's life. I've not been able to cure my so-called superpower, but I have learned to live with it.

Here's a review of the tools and strategies I recommend:

1. Get rid of fluorescent lights.
2. Decrease blue light by limiting screen time.
3. Natural light is your friend.
4. Use low-wattage LEDs in your home.
5. Get yourself spectrum glasses.
6. Buy noise-canceling headphones and/or earbuds.
7. Read printed material rather than on-screen material.

Chapter 13

The Tornado Learning to Multitask with a Brain Injury

I REMEMBER, AS A kid growing up outside of Houston, we would have these tornado watches. Someone on the radio or TV would announce a tornado in the area and tell us to seek shelter. My mom would put me and my sister in the closet, where we would play for a couple hours, coloring in books or reading, trying to ignore the thought of a tornado blowing down our home and whisking us away like Dorothy and Toto.

To this day, I still have nightmares about tornadoes. In some of the nightmares, I am just standing there, watching as a tornado slowly approaches and I am stuck, unable to move.

Maybe you know what it feels like when things are spinning out of control and you don't know what to do. The entire world of responsibility—of bills and to-do lists and work and home life—swirls chaotically around you as you stand, completely frozen, in the center of it.

After a head injury, this feeling can worsen. You might feel as if your head is scattered, as if a tornado has just run through your life, throwing the bits and pieces in every direction and leaving you to clean up the mess. Maybe you've found yourself just sitting static at your desk, staring at nothing, trapped in an immovable state in the middle of a tornado of work or school responsibilities swirling around you. You think, "Why can't I get motivated?"

LIKE A DEER IN THE HEADLIGHTS

Feeling overwhelmed may be new to you after having sustained a head injury. This occurs when your normal motivation drops you like a hot potato, leaving you frustrated, stressed, and bewildered.

You might just sit there, unable to act on the things you need to get done. You might even grab your smartphone and start watching videos of puppies playing in the snow instead of working or studying. Delaying and procrastinating addressing your stack of paperwork, mail, and projects is also common. Tasks that once were easy to accomplish now feel like insurmountable mountains.

BROKEN BATTERY

Higher executive functions are what you need to independently work and study. These brain functions help you solve problems, plan, organize, prioritize, get motivated, learn, speak, think abstractly, spell words, do math in your head, complete projects, and multitask. These brain functions are responsible for your awareness, self-correction, processing speed, and short-term memory. They provide you with the ability to communicate, focus, maintain your attention, manage time effectively, and control your emotions.

These brain functions take a lot of brain energy to power—a resource you are short on while recovering from your brain injury. Like the battery of an old smartphone, an injured brain drains energy stores a lot quicker.

A healthy person wakes up in the morning feeling refreshed. Their mental battery is fully charged. After a brain injury, people often wake up feeling tired. If you're lucky, your brain battery, after a night of sleep, is charged up to 50%.

No Choice but to Persevere

For most people it's not realistic to stop work while their brain is healing. You may be a single-income earner and the primary carrier of your family health benefits. Students studying in college will not always be able to take time off from school. Protecting your brain's energy can help minimize stress at work and lost time at school.

Feeling overwhelmed and stressed when confronted with large work and school projects is common even for people with healthy brains. After a head injury, projects and responsibilities can seem like a scary mission impossible, and you may start to procrastinate and avoid addressing these daunting tasks. Then the tasks start to pile up, making things feel even more insurmountable. In turn you procrastinate more, despite knowing the consequences for things, like paying your bills late.

In Mel Robbins's book *The Five Second Rule*, she explains that "procrastination is not a form of laziness. It has nothing to do with work. It is a need to take a mini stress break. Procrastination is a coping mechanism for stress."[33] She further details why it's important to not beat yourself up for using this coping mechanism. When you do use procrastination to help cope with your stress, you need to be kind and forgive yourself for procrastinating. In her research, she found a paper authored by Dr. Tim Pychyl from Carleton University, showing that students who forgave themselves for procrastinating prior to an exam were less likely to procrastinate for their next exam.[34]

---

[33] Mel Robbins, *The Five Second Rule: Transform Your Life, Work, and Confidence with Everyday Courage* (Brentwood, TN: Savio Republic, 2017), 145.

[34] Michael J.A. Wohl, Timothy A. Pychyl, and Shannon H. Bennett, "I Forgive Myself, Now I Can Study: How Self-Forgiveness for Procrastinating Can Reduce Future Procrastination," *Personality and Individual Differences* 48, no. 7 (May 2010): 803, https://law.utexas.edu/wp-content/uploads/sites/25/Pretend-Paper.pdf.

When you feel this way, put your smartphone down. Grab your journal and a pen. Make a list of the things you need to get done. Look at each item and put them into categories from "urgent" to "can wait until tomorrow." Which item needs to get done now? Which can wait a bit, and which can be done at the end of the day or the next day?

Take each item and break it down to small steps. Every task has a list of small actions that need to be accomplished in order to complete the task. List each small step under the task. Now focus on getting the first small step done. Then take a break until you're ready to move on to the next small task. Continue completing each small step until the task is completed. Once you get some momentum going again, the frozen feeling should subside.

I'm not sure what you do at work, so I will use a pile of mail as an example. Say you have a stack of mail that's been piling up for a while. With your pen and paper, create a list of small steps you will need to complete in order to address this pile of mail. Here's an example:

1. Separate the junk mail from your bills and important mail, creating three smaller piles of mail.
2. Open the individual envelopes.
3. Dispose of the envelopes.
4. Put your bills in order of when the bills are due.
5. Grab your computer or checkbook and put it by the bills.
6. Pay the bills.
7. Put stamps on outgoing mail.
8. Take the mail to the mailbox.

You continue to list these small tasks. Then focus on one small step at a time, taking breaks as you need them.

Remember, don't beat yourself up for feeling frozen or procrastinating. These things are your brain's way of communicating to you that it's feeling overwhelmed. It needs the tasks broken down into smaller steps in order for it to move forward. Looking at your goals and breaking them down into small steps will help you overcome being frozen and help get your motivation going.

Use Alarms

Time management skills are essential for life. However, after a head injury, time management is a whole new ball game. Using alarms on your smartphone is a great way to save brain energy, support your time management skills, and maintain your focus while working or studying.

While working on a project, it takes brain energy to monitor the passing of time. Checking the time repeatedly while working makes you pull your focus away from what you're working on. For someone with a brain injury, this wastes cognitive energy, and that's time that could've been spent focusing on working or studying.

You can use alarms at home to help keep track of time. Alarms can help you remember to take medications, take mental rest breaks, attend meetings, go to appointments, and pick up the kids from school.

Timers are great to help you focus on work, complete tasks in a timely manner, and remind you when it is time to take a break or move on to a new task. Timers can also fill the gaps in your short-term memory by reminding you to turn things off that you have left on, like the sprinklers outside your home or the oven that's roasting your food.

I found that when I was at work, I would feel anxious and start to worry I was going to miss an appointment. I would feel myself constantly looking up anxiously from my work and checking the time. At other times I would be so deeply lost in my work I would completely forget to look up and check the time. Then I realized I was late seeing my next patient. This created a lot of stress for me. I felt as if I was wasting time and energy trying to monitor the passing of time.

When I started setting alarms and timers on my smartphone, I felt a sense of calm. I also used sound alerts, because a ringing or musical noise caught and maintained my attention more than a silent vibrating alarm. I was able to freely dive into the work in front of me. This helped me improve my time management, lowered my stress level, and helped save a little bit of my meager brain energy.

Using alarms and timers helps relieve the mental burden of monitoring time and supports your focus on the task at hand.

STOP BUGGING ME! I'M TRYING TO WORK!

Every day we are inundated with interruptions. Many of them come from your smartphone. Like yelling venders at a carnival, these distractions vie for your attention as you sit and try to focus on important tasks. The distractions are the tornado of to-do lists swirling around in your head. You may have gotten used to these bells, phone vibrations, and window pop-ups, but they cut into your focus and slowly bleed you of your brain's energy.

They also weigh your brain down with oppressive stress. How do you feel when you open your computer or smartphone and see 500 email notifications, 10 text messages, and 20 news feed alerts? Do you feel relaxed or pressured to address those notifications?

These distractions pull you away from your intended plan of getting work done, and instead they drag you down a rabbit hole of shopping for shoes, reading newsletters, searching for vacation destinations, texting funny memes to friends, or watching videos of dogs skateboarding.

Even if you don't have a brain injury, you may still be nodding your head in frustration. Imagine what this tornado does to someone with a brain injury.

To solve this issue, first you need to go into your notification settings on all your smart devices and turn off notifications for unnecessary apps and programs. Also get into the habit of hitting the Do Not Disturb button on your computer every day when you start to study or work. I work with Apple computers, and this button is in the upper-right part of the computer screen.

Then the next thing to do is go through your email and unsubscribe to any email list that's no longer a priority for you. If the email is not from supportive friends and family, unsubscribe. If it's not helping you in your recovery from your brain injury, unsubscribe.

Some email lists allow you to select how often you get an email from its site. If you have a favorite email list, consider cutting back on how frequently it sends you an email. This will take some work, but it will be well worth your time and effort. If this task is too overwhelming, ask a trusted friend or family member to help you unsubscribe from unwanted emails. Over time your email inbox will be more manageable.

Turning off these distractions will improve your focus and attention span, supporting your time management and saving your brain energy for healing.

MULTITASKING IS THE ENEMY OF SANITY

As for multitasking, just let it go. Forget about it. It's highly overrated anyway, and it's a serious myth. Our brains were not designed to multitask.

"The human mind and brain lack the architecture to perform two or more tasks simultaneously," state Drs. Kevin Madore and Anthony Wagner in their article "Multicosts of Multitasking."[35] These researchers further explain that multitasking for people with healthy brains comes at a high cost of increased cognitive demand, decreased efficiency, and increased errors.

Dr. Cheryle Sullivan points out, "It is better to do one thing well, than two or more things poorly."[36] She further recommends "[not] to multitask when needing to remember new information."[37]

Dr. Gail Denton says, "A brain injury reduces brain efficiency, causing us to be able to do only one thing at a time. Gaining focus on the second task takes new energy. Returning to the original task may take another

---

[35] Kevin Madore and Anthony Wagner, "Multicosts of Multitasking," *Cerebrum: The Dana Forum on Brain Science* (April 2019), https://pubmed.ncbi.nlm.nih.gov/32206165.
[36] Cheryle Sullivan, *Brain Injury Survival Kit: 365 Tips, Tools & Tricks to Deal with Cognitive Function Loss* (New York: Demos Health, 2008), 75.
[37] Sullivan, *Brain Injury Survival Kit*, 50.

spurt of energy. Multitask activities may be very taxing or overwhelming at first."[38]

Even though we're not designed to multitask, many of us are expected to in our home and work lives, especially during the pandemic.

People multitask while they are driving, listening to music, or having a conversation with someone. Examples of multitasking might be watching TV and folding laundry. Parents prepare meals while watching small children. You're multitasking when you walk and talk at the same time. For someone recovering from a brain injury, this may be an unrealistic expectation.

Early into your recovery, you may find sharing your focus on two things difficult and fatiguing. You may even find yourself frozen in place between the two tasks.

As your brain heals, you will get better at moving your focus from one task to another, such as walking and talking at the same time or listening to music as you work on your adult coloring. Slowly add these noncomplex tasks, and practice moving your focus between the tasks. As your brain heals and you grow stronger, you may even be able to cook and have a conversation with someone at the same time.

Do stop sharing your focus between two tasks if you feel irritable, become fatigued, get a headache, or start to feel overwhelmed.

Why Memorize What's Already Written Down

Remembering and retaining information is difficult when your brain is healing. Seriously, why memorize something when it is already written down?

A great way to organize information that's difficult to memorize or retain is to put it into a three-ring binder with colorful dividing tabs. If you're

---

[38] Denton, *Brainlash*, 108.

able to compartmentalize the duties of your job, then do so. Try to create a binder for each category of your job. Then take every email, article, or note you have made pertaining to that job duty and organize it in a three-ring binder. Then when you're working on that part of your job, you have all your information in that binder to grab and reference when needed.

At work, I take care of patients with Parkinson's disease. When I started this new job, I was overwhelmed by all the information I need to know to care for these patients. I was also still healing from my brain injury.

So, I created a binder for my patients with Parkinson's disease. Every note or piece of medical information I took was filed in this binder. As I learned how to take care of patients with benign essential tremors or movement disorders, such as Parkinson's disease, I added to my binder. I created several of the same type of binders for patients with other diseases, such as multiple sclerosis and epilepsy. These binders help me take care of my patients and save my brain energy because I didn't have to use the computer to try to find the information I needed. I only had to grab my binder on the subject.

Ask People to Send Emails

Often you will run into co-workers in the hallway, and they'll ask for help with some project or idea. I call these "hallway drive-bys." Whenever you find yourself being sidelined by a hallway drive-by on your way to the bathroom, ask the person to send you an email as a reminder of the discussion or request. That way it will remind you of the by-the-way conversation. It will also allow you time to think, research, or provide the solution or answers that person was seeking from you.

This will help to remind you how to be a supportive team member to co-workers and classmates. It will also lessen your brain load. Attempting to remember drive-by hallway conversations after a brain injury is like trying to swim upstream while tied to a houseboat.

RANDOM BITS AND PIECES

After a brain injury, the world feels like a bunch of random bits and pieces you pick up after a tornado's destruction. It's hard to keep these random things filed in your head. These can be things you need for work or school, but you don't necessarily use them every day, so they won't stick in your head. Maybe you're just too tired all the time to find the energy to commit these things to memory. They could be a person's name or title, a password, or a word you just can't remember how to spell.

For these small random things, use an old-fashion phone or address book to help organize these small memory items in a way that you can reference on the go. These paper phone or address books have letter tabs marking the pages inside of them. I recommend getting a small one that will fit in your pocket.

Use the letter tabs inside the address books to organize bits and pieces of information your brain just doesn't want to remember. Then when you need that information, you just go to the letter and look at those pages. For example, you might not be able to remember the name of the woman who helps you with computer training. You might put her name under *I* for IT specialist. On the page you would keep her name, contact information, or any personal information she has shared with you, like her beloved dog's name. Before a meeting with her, you can pull out your phone book and glance at her information to remind you.

I've also heard of a lawyer who had a brain injury. After his injury, he struggled to remember people's names, titles, and professions. So, he used three-by-five-inch index cards. He would write these people's information down on the card, and when he had a meeting with them, he would tuck their card in his pocket. He would pull out the card and refresh his memory as he arrived at the meeting and glance at it as needed during the meeting.

I recommend going low tech with support strategies early in your recovery. As your brain heals and brain energy expands, switching to a smart device for memory strategies would be reasonable.

CHECKOFF LIST AND ROUTINE

Early into your recovery, you may need to use checkoff lists as an external memory tool until your brain has the steps solidified into a routine.

I used checkoff lists the first year of my recovery. I wrote my checkoff list in a small pocketbook I kept in my back pocket. I used these checkoff lists to remember all the things I needed to pack for work and to remember when caring for my patients.

You can use a checkoff list to remember important steps in a task until completing the task becomes an automatic routine.

STOP TRYING TO ACCOMPLISH THE IMPOSSIBLE

Renée Montagne and Chana Joffe-Walt reported in February 2009 during National Public Radio's *Morning Edition* that workers were hearing the phrase "do more with less."[39]

If your job expects blood out of beets, realize that you need to have realistic expectations. Don't beat yourself up if you cannot keep up with your work. The reasons that you're unable to keep up and perform at the standard you expect of yourself may not solely be due to your brain injury.

Remember to look around you. Are your fellow students and co-workers looking tired, frazzled, and stressed? Are they complaining of headaches and not being able to keep up with their work demands too? Are you seeing them missing days at work or skipping class? Then this tells you that you and your brain are being expected to accomplish an impossible workload. If your co-workers are struggling to keep up, then don't expect you and your healing brain to keep up either. Don't let the delusional demands of your instructors or manager stress you out.

---

[39] Renée Montagne and Chana Joffe-Walt, "Workplace Refrain: Do More with Less," *Morning Edition*, NPR, February 26, 2009, https://www.npr.org/templates/story/story.php?storyId=101177718.

Do the best job you can do. Work within the limits of your and your brain's abilities. Let go of meeting your own personal work standards that you held prior to your head injury. Remember, your top priorities are to do your best and to be kind to yourself and your brain.

RECAP

Getting control of your tornado of to-do lists and responsibilities is a hard enough task for someone without a brain injury. For people like you and me, it may seem like a near-impossible task. But trust me, it can be done. You will just need to develop new routines and strategies to help you regain control.

Here's a review of the things you can do:

1. Protect your focus. Have co-workers use an electronic messaging tool instead of meeting you at your desk.
2. Avoid multitasking.
3. Use low-tech tools like binders, writing pads, or address books to replace your memory until it is trustworthy again.
4. Use checkoff lists until tasks are routine.
5. Use smart devices to support your memory only after your cognitive stamina and tolerance of blue light increases.

Chapter 14

Don't Break Your Brain—
Give It a Brain Break

REMEMBER WHEN YOU WERE in kindergarten and how nap time was scheduled in the middle of the day? Back in my day, everyone had to stop playing, sit quietly, drink their milk, and eat their graham crackers. Then you went to your cubbyhole, got your fluffy, soft blanket, laid it on the floor, and took a nap.

It turns out that everything we needed to learn, we learned in kindergarten. Researchers have touted the benefits of breaks for both employees and students—but they're especially crucial for those with head trauma. In her book, *Mild Traumatic Brain Injury: The Guidebook*, Mary Lou Acimovic explains, "When it comes to maintaining a sustainable level of productivity throughout the day, taking hourly 'Brain Breaks' is one of the best things anyone with a mild TBI can do."[40] Taking brain breaks intermittently throughout your day can make a full day of work or school achievable.

---

[40] Acimovic, *Mild Traumatic Brain Injury*, 227.

WHAT IS A BRAIN BREAK?

Brain breaks can be as brief as a few seconds of looking away from your computer. However, they can also be as long as a day or a week. Sometimes you need to give your brain a little vacation by taking some time off from school or work. We call these mental health days.

After a head injury, it's recommended to take frequent breaks while working or studying. Alan Hedge, in his article *"Workstation Ergonomics: Take a Break!,"* shares the following different types of breaks people should incorporate into their schedules: eye breaks, rest breaks, and exercise breaks.[41]

Here are a few different breaks you'll want to consider throughout your day:

- **Eye breaks:** These are recommended for people with healthy brains. It's best to take an eye break every 15 minutes. This is a micro break and requires very little from you. All you need to do is simply look away from your computer for one to two minutes. Try looking out the window, or if you don't have a window, look at something at least 20 feet away.

- **Rest breaks:** Rest breaks are recommended every 30 to 60 minutes. This type of break forces you to get up and walk around, get a beverage, use the restroom, or stretch. For these breaks you need to get up and move. Walk away from your work or study materials. Doing so combats fatigue, overuse injuries, and stiff muscles.

- **Exercise breaks:** These are when you do some gentle stretching or go for a short walk. These breaks should be taken every one to two hours, even for healthy people. These breaks promote emotional health, improve blood circulation, and stimulate productivity and creativity.

---

[41] Alan Hedge, "Workstation Ergonomics: Take a Break!," Spine Universe, September 3, 2019, https://www.spineuniverse.com/wellness/ergonomics/workstation-ergonomics-take-break.

Your brain energy and stamina will dictate how frequently you need to take these various breaks. It can be difficult incorporating breaks into your schedule, especially if you're not used to them. This is why it's best to set a timer to remind you when to take a break.

Taking breaks will support your brain's healing and your ability to make it through a work or school day. Brain breaks will help you sustain control of your emotions and promote positive interactions with others. Taking intermittent breaks will power up your productivity and support your focus and creativity.

Intermittent brief breaks from work and study are important for healthy children and adults but even more so for people with brain injuries. Taking brain breaks after a head injury is imperative for maintaining emotional stability and productivity, preventing mistakes in school, and avoiding dangerous errors at work. (Yes, we're not that much different from a kindergartener. It takes a lot of energy to filter out the world, and we need the rest too.)

I'm Tired of Resting

Establishing the habit of taking brain breaks can be difficult for some. You might think at times you can't take a break, or you may worry you'll be judged as lazy. You also may just want to power through your exhaustion. When you have a brain injury, these thoughts will come back to haunt you.

You might also be like me. My curiosity, passion, and love for learning far exceeds my cognitive brain-energy capacity. Sometimes when it's time for me to take a break, I feel like a pouting toddler who has been told to go to her room for nap time. I scream in my head like a little kid, "Nooooooo! I want to keep reading!"

Having to take breaks is frustrating and can be downright depressing. But as time passes and your brain heals, your brain will eventually share more of its energy with you.

Don't Have a Toddler Tantrum

It's not wise to skip brain breaks. Mary Lou Acimovic explains in her book, *Mild Traumatic Brain Injury: The Guidebook*, "You need to let go of using your work lunch or school breaks to hang out with friends or colleagues, run errands, or to make phone calls. After a head injury there should also be no working through lunch or straight through without taking a break."[42] These breaks are essential to allow your brain to rest and recoup.

If you skip taking breaks, you're risking the chance of having a meltdown in front of your colleagues. In *Brainlash: Maximize Your Recovery from Mild Brain Injury*, Dr. Gail Denton says, "With brain injury, you may not be able to modulate your emotional body because you simply do not have the energy to do so."[43] It's best to take your breaks before you get tired. Remember, your brain needs energy to heal. It's not going to put up with you burning it out.

Pushing your brain beyond its threshold will also land you in the penalty box of recovery regression. This is not a good place to be.

Mild regression in your recovery is inevitable while you find balance between supporting your healing, getting stronger, and overdoing it because you have a life to live. Choosing to go to a social gathering or drive out of town may cause you to regress in your recovery. A day of quiet and a nap can help restore you to your recovery baseline.

However, if you insist on not listening and not obeying your brain's signals that it needs a break, and you demand too much from it, your brain will smack you down like an unwanted mosquito. You'll feel as if you have gone back to the first weeks after your head injury, functioning as if you're at square one. Most likely this will cause you to experience the return of symptoms such as headaches, mood swings, slower processing of even basic information, poor memory recall, dizziness, and unbelievable exhaustion. It's also possible that you'll need to spend several days sleeping

---

[42] Acimovic, *Mild Traumatic Brain Injury*, 173.
[43] Denton, *Brainlash*, 36.

just to recover, and you will be back on your couch, exhausted and feeling like a loser.

Measuring and Protecting Your Brain's Stamina

As your brain recovers, it will have a limited amount of cognitive stamina.

To measure your brain stamina, set a timer and start reading or working on a computer. When your focus breaks, your eyes grow tired, or your concentration wanes, check the timer and note the time. This is when your brain will need a break.

It's best to take a break before you're tired, just like it is best to get kindergartners to take a nap before they start throwing a tantrum. If you notice that you're irritable, or any of the other symptoms, take a break. Now that you know when to take a break and how often, set a reminder alarm.

At least every three to six months, repeat this test, measuring your brain stamina on various tasks of reading, computer work, or working on projects. As your brain heals, these time frames should expand.

I'll Take a Side of Naptime with My Salad

Oh boy, this is a tough strategy to implement for most people. Employers frown on sleeping on the job, but sleep researchers' findings show naps help healthy employees improve their performance.[44]

If possible, you should spend your lunch break laying down and taking a 20-minute nap. This will help you get through the other half of the day and perform at your best. At a minimum, I recommend laying back and closing your eyes during your lunch. Getting your feet on the same level as your head can be restorative to your mind and body. Even if you can only

---

[44] Mark Mattei, "Power Napping on the Job: It May Help Your Company Save Money," Sleep Advisor, https://www.sleepadvisor.org/sleeping-at-work/.

put your feet up on your desk and lean back in your chair and shut your eyes, do it. Another rejuvenating position is laying on a yoga mat with a pillow behind your head while your feet and knees rest on a chair.

Dr. Matthew Walker explains in his book, *Why We Sleep*, that humans are supposed to sleep in a biphasic pattern: our natural sleep pattern should be sleeping at night for seven to nine hours and then taking a 30- to 60-minute nap in the afternoon.[45]

So people with healthy brains who have large energy reserves are by nature programmed for an afternoon siesta. This explains the normal after-lunch drowsiness you see with your co-workers in late meetings and classmates in afternoon classes.

Now imagine how strong that pull for an afternoon nap is for the person who has a brain injury and a small amount of brain energy reserved. Let me tell you, that pull to sleep in the afternoon is nothing like normal sleepiness. It's an overwhelming tsunami wave that crashes down on you.

Unfortunately, I did not have a quiet space to put my feet up, close my eyes, and relax at my work. So, I would go out to my car and lay down in the back seat. Keep in mind that it's not safe for people to sleep in their cars. I do not recommend it for others. However, I was so tired by lunchtime, I did not care. It would feel as if I were barely able to walk a straight line while going to my car because I would be dizzy with exhaustion. Often I would crawl in the back seat of my car, lock the doors, drop my head down and check out, like a terminated cyborg. My alarm clock would wake me up, and I would find my face laying in a pool of my drool.

Since I was working 40-plus hours a week, this was something I had to do to get through the day. I kept a blanket and pillows in my car for my naps.

No one wants to work with a person who looks like a drowned raccoon, so before I would go into the office, I would brush my skewed hair and

---

[45] Matthew Walker, *Why We Sleep: Unlocking the Power of Sleep and Dreams* (New York: Scribner, 2017), 17–19.

fix my smeared mascara and eye liner with the extra makeup and comb I kept in my car.

Over time as my brain healed, I was able to skip my lunch break naps. But I still go out to my car for quiet time so I can relax a little and close my eyes if needed.

There are some companies that recognize that well-rested employees are more alert, productive, and creative. These companies know this equates to profits for their bottom line. Nike and Google are two that provide their employees with nap rooms.

Dr. Matthew Walker further shares that "NASA redefined the science of sleeping on the job for the benefit of their astronauts. They discovered that naps as short as 26 minutes in length still offered a 34% improvement in task performance and more than a 50% improvement increase in overall alertness."[46]

It's too bad that more employers don't offer this to their employees.

So, if you can, have a side of a nap with your salad at lunch. Your brain will reward you with a bit more cognitive energy and stamina to get you through the other half of your day.

Be Strategic with Vacation, Mental Health, and Sick Days

People with healthy brains need mental health days, and people who have head injuries require them. A mental health day is time away from work when you simply need a mental break.

K. Wong, A. Chan, and S. C. Ngan reported in their article "The Effect of Long Working Hours and Overtime on Occupational Health: A Meta-Analysis of Evidence from 1998 to 2018," "that employees working long hours were vulnerable to suffering from diverse types of occupational

---

[46] Walker, *Why We Sleep*, 305.

health problem."[47] People, especially women working 40-plus hours a week, can put their mental health at risk.

When you have a brain injury, emotional stress is a trigger that will drain your energy and worsen brain injury symptoms. If you experience emotional stress on top of your regular day-to-day stress, this additional stress has the potential to cause you to regress in your recovery.

A mental health day may be needed when stress accumulates, and you cannot push through another work or school day. If you do not rest and stay home, you may feel like hitting someone over the head with a chair. With that thought in mind, for everyone else's safety, just take a mental health day.

Some work environments are demanding. Depending on your work demands and environment, taking a mental health day may not be a realistic expectation—let alone for a person with a brain injury. Jim Harter and Vipula Gandhi, in their article "7 Things We Learned About U.S. and Canadian Employees in 2020," reported "Gallup's *State of the Global Workplace: 2021 Report* found that workers in the U.S. and Canada reported the highest rate of daily stress in the world during 2020."[48]

If your job is too demanding, you should strongly consider looking for another one.

Here are some common signs that you need a mental health day:

- You feel irritable, short-tempered, emotionally edgy, angry, or stressed, and short breaks don't help.
- Fatigue is affecting your alertness and thinking.

---

[47] K. Wong, A. H. S. Chan, and S. C. Ngan, "The Effect of Long Working Hours and Overtime on Occupational Health: A Meta-Analysis of Evidence from 1998 to 2018," *International Journal of Environmental Research and Public Health* 16, no. 12 (June 2019): 2102, https://doi.org/10.3390/ijerph16122102.

[48] Jim Harter and Vipula Gandhi, "7 Things We Learned About U.S. and Canadian Employees in 2020," Gallup, June 15, 2021, https://www.gallup.com/workplace/350123/united-states-canada-workplace-trends.aspx.

- You don't believe you can work safely.
- You've missed sleep, had a sleepless night, or are sleep deprived.
- You're feeling burned out.
- You're taking work frustrations personally.
- You have dizziness or difficulty with your balance.
- Your brain injury symptoms are returning or worsening.
- You have or are recovering from a migraine headache or post-concussive headache.

On your mental health day, take care of your brain. First replenish any missed sleep. Go to bed early and wake up late. Allow your brain to sleep as long as it needs to. When you're ready to get out of bed, eat healthy foods during your meals and drink lots of fluids.

Spend some time doing mindful thinking. Spend time outside, go on a walk, watch the sunset, practice yoga, work on adult coloring or a favorite craft project. Don't work on a to-do list unless it will help relieve your stress if you get some things done. Still, do simple, easy tasks.

Most employers frown on taking mental health days or don't offer them. If this is the case at your place of employment, you may need to be strategic about your vacation and sick days.

One of my patients knows that she cannot work more than two to three weeks without taking a mental health day. If she does, she has said, "I will lose my shit and go off at the mouth and get fired." So, she plans days off by strategically requesting a day off every two to three weeks. If she does not have the vacation time, she calls in sick and uses her sick time. She says, "This is how I keep my job."

If your employer does not offer or support mental health days, don't feel obligated to share why you need the time off or why you had a sick day. If you're unable to work part time, you should use your time-off benefits wisely. To avoid having to call in sick after you have reached your mental or physical stress limits, consider planning days off in advance, like my patient does.

Keep track in your calendar of how long you can go between mental health days, and once you know, you can plan days off in advance. You can then request the time off. A planned day off is also better for you because it helps you look forward to that three-day weekend. It can be a big motivator to get you through the days prior to that time off. Giving your employer advance notice of needed time off will also keep you off the hot seat and avoid an attendance evaluation with a mean manager.

You may have to forgo your normal weeklong vacations in order to spread your time-off days to make this work. This can be a real bummer of a decision to make. Hopefully you will only have to do this until your brain heals.

THESE BOOTS ARE MADE FOR WALKING

If you're at work or school and find yourself feeling frozen, overwhelmed, emotional, or unable to start a task, the best thing to do is get up and walk away from your desk. Do not stay seated, attempt to continue to work, or suppress these feelings. This will worsen your symptoms and affect your work performance. Not addressing these issues immediately may lead you to snap at a co-worker or classmate.

This signal is your brain's attempt to communicate with you that you need to take a time-out. Listen to what your brain is telling you. Grab your brain recovery journal and get outside or walk away for a little bit.

These are what Dr. Cheryle Sullivan calls "cognitive breaks."[49] Find a calming location away from your desk that's quiet and has minimal foot traffic. Nature is perfect for this, even if it's just a break area outside.

If you can't walk out of your work area, consider going to the restroom. In the restroom, if possible, turn off the lights or sit in a stall with your eyes closed. Once away from your desk in a quieter place, concentrate on taking several slow, deep breaths. When you feel your body and mind relax, this

---

[49] Sullivan, *Brain Injury Survival Kit*, 2.

is the time to look back on those feelings you were having and what may have caused them. Was there too much light and sound? When was the last time you ate? Did the task you were working on feel too big for you to accomplish?

What strategies do you need to employ to address these feelings? Make notes to reflect on later in your journal. When you feel ready, go back to your desk. The key here is to not be afraid to just walk away.

RECAP

1. Naptime is not just for kids.
2. After a head injury, take frequent breaks while working or studying.
3. Use a timer to remind you to take a break.
4. It's best to take a brain break before you're tired.
5. Walk away from working or studying when you start to feel emotionally stressed or frustrated.
6. Brain breaks are best taken in a non-stimulating, quiet space.
7. Always choose a mental health day over being fired.

While you're healing, these brain breaks may need to be taken more frequently until your brain-energy reserves and stamina increase. However, keep in mind that even healthy brains need frequent breaks too. So be kind to your brain as it heals and grows stronger and give it some breaks.

Chapter 15

Getting Off on the Wrong Foot
I'm Late, I'm Late, for a Very Important Date!

AFTER A HEAD INJURY, you may find yourself perpetually late to appointments and social engagements, even if you're the type of person who usually arrives early. Now when you try to make it to an appointment, you might find yourself moving in slow motion, and the time you thought you had to get ready has been sucked up in a vortex.

The ability to sense the passing of time, calculate how long it will take you to get ready, and travel to your destination is a higher executive function of our brains that most people take for granted. Remember, higher executive functions take a lot of energy to power, and that's energy injured brains don't have. In her book, *Mild Traumatic Brain Injury: The Guidebook*, Mary Lou Acimovic explains this is an "adult skill that is often lost after a head injury."[50]

Not having to adult is awesome, but not being able to adult sucks. Before my head injury, I could easily calculate how much time it would take

---

⁵⁰ Acimovic, *Mild Traumatic Brain Injury*, 36.

to get ready and travel to social gatherings. I would rarely have to glance at a clock as I headed out the door.

Figuring out how to be on time after my head injury was a serious struggle of one embarrassing failure after another. No matter how hard I tried, I could not get my brain around the concept of how much time I needed to arrive at my planned engagement. I was never on time and was always getting off on the wrong foot.

Don't Get Caught Out in the Rain without an Umbrella

One of my favorite life adventures was living in Portland, Oregon. When I lived there, I was surprised at how quickly the weather could change. You could walk into Powell's bookstore, and the sun would be shining, but 10 minutes later while standing in line to purchase your books, you might look out and see a downpour. If you did not want to brave the buckets of rain, you could opt to grab a cup of warm coffee in the bookstore's cozy café, and by the time you turned to leave the coffee counter, the rain may have subsided to a gentle drizzle. Then, as you drove home, the sun would peek through the clouds.

These weather changes were so notorious that the locals would say, "If you don't like the weather, just wait five minutes and it will change." As such, I learned it was best to always have an umbrella in my car or purse.

When I moved back to California, I kept this habit of keeping an umbrella all year long in my car. My friends would always be surprised to see I had an umbrella ready whenever it rained. I was always ready.

Being caught in pouring rain without an umbrella is no fun, which is why it's always best to be prepared for what may come your way. This is even more essential when you're recovering from a head injury.

One of the things you can do to work around rough mornings is to prepare your morning routine the night before. You may be able to set everything up so that all you have to do is crawl out of bed, press a couple buttons, grab your lunch out of the fridge, and head out the door.

If you have a programable coffee maker, set it up the night before. There is nothing like waking up to the smell of coffee. All this preparation will create a morning with minimal decision-making, saving your brain's energy for work that actually matters. You may even want to keep an umbrella in the car.

BEING LATE DRAINS YOUR SHORT SUPPLY OF ENERGY

One of the top brain-energy drainers is emotional stress, and there's nothing more distressing than starting your day out on the wrong foot. You will find yourself arriving to work or school late and already exhausted, irritated, and stressed out as soon as your day begins.

After a head injury, your mornings are going to totally suck. It's going to feel as if even more chaos has been thrown into your life, but you're just going to have to figure out a way around it because it's expected that employees and students arrive prepared and on time.

In addition to preparing as much as you can the night before, you may want to have a checkoff list that you reference as you get ready for the next day. Recheck it before leaving your home. Let the list do the thinking for you.

Early into my recovery, my checkoff lists kept me from forgetting the steps I needed to take to get ready for the next day. I had to use these checkoff lists for over a year. Today I still use a checkoff list whenever my routine is changed.

NO MANIC MONDAYS

The biggest thing that can deter you from wanting to get out of your warm, cozy bed is having to figure out what you're going to wear for the day. Making these decisions in the morning can also cause you to run late. That's why you should select your clothes the night before.

First, check the weather prior to selecting your outfit. This will help you pick clothes you will be comfortable in for the next day. You don't want to be caught wearing your spring dress on a rainy day. Once you have the entire outfit, hang it all together in your bathroom.

Include not only your outfit but also undergarments, socks, shoes, and accessories. The goal is to not leave any fashion decisions for the next morning, so you won't burn up your brain energy.

In the morning, stick to a routine when getting dressed and caring for your hygiene. Try doing everything in the same order every morning: brush teeth, get dressed, do hair, etc. Sticking to that routine will help you not spend brain energy on having to remember if you did everything before leaving the bathroom.

If needed, use another checkoff list that you keep in your bathroom until you have your routine down pat in an automatic mode.

PACK YOUR BAGS

The night before, make sure everything you need for work or school is packed in your bags, like your wallet, headphones, books, laptop, phone charger, and dark glasses. Then place your bags on the kitchen counter to grab in the morning.

Also pack food you plan to eat while you're away from home. Things that don't need to be refrigerated should go in your work bag. Put refrigerated food in to-go containers so they're ready for you to grab in the morning. I store my food in to-go containers on the weekend so they're all ready for me to grab throughout the week. Then place refrigerated items in the same spot or drawer in the refrigerator. So, when you look in that spot in the morning, the food will be there to remind you to pack your lunch in the cooler.

When you pack everything in your car, pack them together. That will help you to grab everything when you exit your car. You don't want to forget a bag you put behind your car seat or in the trunk.

Two Are Better Than One

Another option for making sure you don't leave the house without forgetting things is buying duplicate items. These are items that are easy to forget when you are in a rush. For instance, having an extra phone charger at work comes in handy. If you forget to brush your teeth or do your daily hygiene routine, having back-up deodorant, a toothbrush, and toothpaste in your bag or at work will help ease some of your morning stress. Also, consider keeping cash in your car in case you leave your wallet at home.

I used to dread the day I would forget my noise-canceling headphones or dark glasses at home. The thought of going through a day at work without them would send me into a panic. I couldn't stand feeling this way and risking not being able to safely focus on my patient care while at work. So, I decided to invest in multiple pairs of light-blocking glasses and two sets of noise-canceling earbuds and headphones.

I leave one set at work and keep the other set at home. This relieved some of my mental stress. For me, two was better than one.

Planning Your Day

Your brain will have the most energy at the beginning of the day. As the day progresses, your energy will dwindle down like an old cell phone battery with no option for a recharge. Plan your toughest tasks at the beginning of the day when you have the most brain energy. Save your easier tasks, like putting away your laundry, for the end of the day.

If something pops up during your day that makes you feel overwhelmed, or you're just too tired to give it the attention it needs, set the task aside for the next day and plan to work on it first thing in the morning.

How to Arrive on Time

A few months after my head injury, after racking my brain, I finally was able to find a system that worked for me. I still use this strategy today when I need to travel out of town, go to a new place, or disrupt my normal routine. Hopefully these tips I've learned will work for you too.

I call my time management strategy a reverse-time list. I grab a piece of paper and pen and write at the top the time I need to be at the destination. Then I go to Google Maps to see the time it will take to travel from my home to my destination. I then add 15 to 30 minutes for traffic and 10 minutes to find parking.

Early into my recovery, I doubled the time I thought it would take me to get ready. If I thought it would take me a half hour, I would give myself one hour to get ready. Then I would work the schedule down the list, marking the time I needed to start the next step to get out of my home on time.

I would do this the night before the appointment and set reminder alarms on my smartphone to measure the passing of time for my brain. As I got ready, I would glance at my list and the time to see that I was on schedule.

This is an example of what a reverse-time list would look like:

- Arrive at work, 8:30 a.m.
- Exit my car (15 minutes), 8:15 a.m.
- Park car (10 minutes), 8:05 a.m.
- Leave to travel (40 minutes plus a 15-minute cushion), 7:10 a.m.
- Pack up car, (15 minutes) 6:55 a.m.
- Make coffee and pack lunch, (30 minutes) 6:25 a.m.
- Get ready, (25 minutes) 6 a.m.
- Set alarm clock to wake up, (10 minutest to wake up) 5:50 a.m.

This was the only way I could figure out how to be on time to my planned destinations, like an adult should. I hope it helps you.

RECAP

Getting organized the night before will ensure you start the day on the right foot, safely, prepared, and on time. Using these strategies will help you avoid feeling overwhelmed and save your brain energy for your plans for the day. Perhaps now you will never get caught in the rain without an umbrella.

Use these steps when preparing the night before:

1. Create a reverse-time list.
2. Choose your clothes.
3. Make your lunch.
4. Prep the coffee machine.
5. Pack your bags.
6. Make a morning routine checkoff list.

Chapter 16
Managing Your To-Do List: I'm Sorry. What Memory?

THINK OF YOUR BRAIN like a computer. It has a certain amount of bandwidth, memory, storage, and RAM. It responds quickly to your requests and operates smoothly between applications and the internet. Your brain is able to keep track of things you need to get done like grocery shop, pay bills, answer emails, finish a work project, clean out the garage, walk the dog, pick up the kids from school, and make dinner. The memory can retain lists that seemingly go on and on.

Well, after your head injury, you may notice that your computer no longer works as well, almost as if you've dropped it.

The next few days your computer turns on, but it's slower to respond when switching apps. When you go to the internet, it says the page cannot be found, or it takes you to pages that aren't relevant to your search word.

A few weeks go by, and you notice when you click to save a project that the file is deleted or that your project is stored in the hard drive under some unknown file, which you are unable to retrieve. At this point, you may decide it's time to buy a new computer.

Unfortunately, you cannot buy a new brain.

EXTERNAL MEMORY SYSTEMS

As we all know, highly productive people who accomplish goals use to-do lists in their personal and professional lives. You may have been one of these people yourself prior to your head injury. But after a head injury, you may find having and maintaining a to-do list and calendar is crucial to your life, work, or study. Mary Lou Acimovic says, in her book, *Mild Traumatic Brain Injury: The Guidebook,* "Act as if you have no memory. Adopt an external system."[51] This external system—a.k.a. a to-do list for your life—replaces your brain's memory and allows it to heal.

On good days, your memory may seem to work as it used to. Oh, but wait. Sit back and grab some popcorn when emotional stress, fatigue, a terrible headache, a bad night of sleep, or a change in your routine happens. Your memory will leave you hanging in the wind. Sometimes it works, and sometimes it doesn't.

You may forget to go to doctor appointments, to pick up your kids from school, or even to turn off the oven. I often forgot to go to appointments, to feed my pets, and to pay bills. Thank goodness my pets had better memories than I did. My brain's memory even led me to forget to turn off a water hose with a stop-spray nozzle. Fortunately, the hose exploded before the pipes in the house! My husband found the exploded mess after finding water draining from our house into the street.

If you're ever going to get back to some semblance of "normalcy," whatever that means, you will need to learn or relearn how to effectively manage a to-do list. A to-do list is different from a checkoff list discussed in the previous chapter. A checkoff list *is* an external system, but it helps you remember steps to take to complete a routine task, like getting ready

---

[51] Acimovic, *Mild Traumatic Brain Injury,* 171.

and dressed for work. You use these until you have your routine down pat in an automatic mode. A to-do list is to help you remember the things you want to accomplish during the day, the week, or the next hour, such as pay bills or fold the laundry.

Here are the things you will need for this chapter:

- A notebook for your home recovery journal
- A notebook for your work or school recovery journal
- A month-at-a-glance calendar
- A small pocket-size notebook
- Sticky notes
- Your favorite pen

WHY WASTE BRAIN ENERGY ON SOMETHING THAT CAN BE WRITTEN DOWN?

The benefit of to-do lists is that they help shift your mental load from your brain onto paper.

Before your head injury, you may have been able to keep some smaller items stored in your head while your to-do list contained complex tasks and larger projects. Now you may realize managing a to-do list along with a calendar is too much.

Do you hear that? That's the sound of your computer fan working on overdrive because you're trying to store too much information in your head. If you're not careful, your computer might crash.

Why waste brain energy on something that can be written down? Think of a to-do list as downloading some of your memory onto an external hard drive to free up some of the available space and energy in your brain. Once you put down the things you're trying to keep memorized in your head onto paper, you may feel a relief from the stressful strain of trying to hold on tightly to those thoughts.

SLOTH MODE

For most people with a head injury, expecting your brain to sustain multiple thoughts and plans at once is unreasonable. Staying organized, managing time wisely, and being productive is a serious struggle even for people with healthy brains.

Memory is a complicated process. This process demands a lot of energy. Think about a computer with a ton of tabs open. Although in the past we may have been able to manage all those different tasks, now those tabs are slowing us down, making our hard drive work overtime, and occasionally causing our computer to crash.

This can leave you feeling frustrated, fatigued, lazy, or stupid. You are none of these things. You just have a brain injury.

GOAL: HOW TO MANAGE A TO-DO LIST AFTER A BRAIN INJURY

Managing a to-do list is a complex task. Do not expect to manage a to-do list early into your recovery. A good indicator that you're ready to manage a to-do list is when you feel comfortable completing your routine daily checkoff lists. It's also a good idea to practice managing to-do lists prior to returning to work and school.

Your initial to-do list should be short with noncomplex undertakings. Noncomplex tasks do not require critical thinking, such as simple or repetitive tasks. They're familiar tasks you would normally do while on "autopilot." But after your brain injury, they may require some attention and focus. These include the following:

- Folding laundry
- Vacuuming
- Sweeping a floor
- Hand washing dishes

- Putting clothes away
- Cleaning out a drawer
- Watering outside plants
- Raking leaves
- Making a sandwich

Complex tasks require concentration, critical thinking, abstract thought, working memory, planning, decision-making, and execution. Below are examples of complex tasks:

- Completing paperwork
- Reading and writing
- Learning something new
- Studying for a test
- Cooking
- Managing bills
- Creating a budget
- Planning a party
- Making a call to the insurance company or bank
- Driving
- Traveling
- Hiring someone for a house repair
- Computer work

As your brain heals, slowly increase the number of noncomplex undertakings, such as emptying the dishwasher, and add one complex assignment, such as making an important call, completing paperwork, or responding to emails.

It can be difficult at first for some to keep and follow a to-do list. Some of my patients say they stopped keeping to-do lists because they kept losing the list. Also, if not managed appropriately, your to-do list can become too long and overwhelming.

How to Keep Track of and Maintain Your To-Do List

To keep from losing your to-do list, you need to keep the list in the same place. Some people keep a to-do list and family calendar on a shared board in the kitchen.

What worked best for me is keeping my to-do list in my recovery journal. This kept me from losing it, and since I always kept my journal with me, my to-do list was always within reach.

How do you keep from losing the little items you used to keep on your mental list? Leo Babauta, the author of *Zen to Done: The Ultimate Simple Productivity System*, recommends creating a habit he calls "collect."[52] With this habit, Leo suggests always keeping a small notebook or stack of index cards with you. I preferred a small notebook, because the pages are kept together and were less likely to be separated and lost. Your little notebook should be small enough to fit in your pocket and keep with you wherever you go. I kept mine in my back pocket with a pen.

This small notebook replaces your brain's shoddy memory process and becomes your working memory. When you think of something or see something that needs to be done, grab your notebook and write it down immediately. Then when you're sitting down with your head injury journal, write these things down on your main to-do list.

You can do the same thing with a grocery list. Any time you think of something you need to buy at the grocery store, write it down quickly before it's gone.

Create Your Main To-Do List

As you go through the day, write things you want to remember, like random

---

[52] Leo Babauta, *Zen to Done: The Ultimate Simple Productivity System* (Salt Lake City: Waking Lion Press, 2011), 5.

thoughts, plans, and chores, in your pocket notebook. Remember to always keep the pocket notebook with you. Later write these items on your main to-do list in your recovery journal.

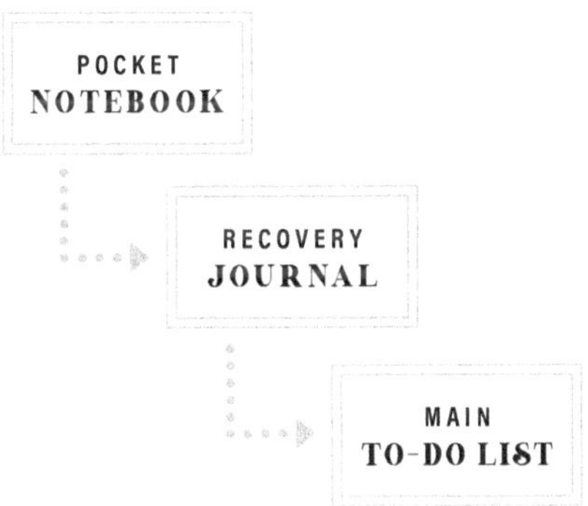

How to Organize and Manage Your To-Do List

Your to-do list is a tool that is supposed to support your memory, focus, and motivation. However, if not managed correctly, a to-do list can turn into a long, chaotic, anxiety-causing monster of torture. There are many books and resources on the internet on how to manage to-do lists. You may be familiar with Stephen Covey's *7 Habits of Highly Effective People* and his way of managing to-do lists. He's a highly productive, highly motivated go-getter. He also does not have a brain injury.

Prior to my head injury, I managed my to-do lists based on Stephen Covey's recommendations. Alas, after my head injury this system was just too complex for me, and I soon found myself staring frozen at my to-do lists.

I then found Leo Babauta's *Zen to Done* book, which is also available on Audible. I was looking for tools to help with my productivity and for ways to simplify my life. This turned out to be a great system for me. I encourage you to follow or develop a system that works best for you.

CREATING CATEGORIES AND A SOMEDAY LIST

Leo Babauta's method centers on one specific method: don't place all your tasks on one huge, never-ending to-do list.[53] A to-do list should be small. You do this by placing the tasks you want to remember and accomplish into separate categories.

First you should look at your list of tasks. Don't forget to ask for help with your list if you need it. Now while looking at this list, start to separate tasks that you must do from those you want to do. For example, paying bills goes under the must-do list and working on a puzzle would go on a want-to-do list.

Now you have your must-do list and your want-to-do list. Further separate these tasks into things that need to be done this month and things that can wait.

Look for tasks that can wait until "someday." For me a someday list took a lot of stress off my mind. Things you can put on your someday list are goals, plans, and personal projects that you may not be able to do while recovering. These are things you do not want to forget to do someday when you are stronger. For example, you probably don't need to get your house painted this month or to clean out and organize your garage this weekend.

When you return to work or school, you will need to create a to-do list for home and one for work or school. I recommend keeping your home to-do list in your recovery journal and your work or school to-do list in your work or school recovery journals.

After you have your separated home and work or school to-do lists, you need to sit down and look at your tasks. Start to separate the tasks into smaller categories. For example, a home to-do list may have categories such as grocery list, finances, yard chores, household items that need restocking, this month's birthdays, errands, DIY projects, or household repairs.

---

[53] Babauta, *Zen to Done*, 29-30.

Work or school to-do list categories could be things you need to get done while at your computer, continuing education, training classes, administrative paperwork, phone calls, projects, and professional goals.

With this said, you don't want a ton of tiny to-do lists either, because that can be overwhelming too. You will need to find the balance that works best for you. I like creating categories of tasks. One list category could be a computer list. Under this category you list all the things you need to do while on the computer, such as emails to write, bills to pay, or topics you want to research on the internet.

How to Actually Do Things on Your To-Do List

After you have your main list separated into categories, you will use them as a reference when planning your days in the week. When starting to use a to-do list, plan to get to work on one complex task with one to two non-complex tasks a day. If you can complete your daily goals without being exhausted or irritable, then start adding on more tasks. This has the added benefit of measuring how well your brain is healing.

Leo Babauta recommends in his book, *Zen to Done: The Ultimate Simple Productivity System*, "Each day create a list of 1–3 most important tasks."[54] So Leo Babauta does not recommend even for people with healthy brains to demand of themselves more than three complex tasks in a day. As your brain is healing, a more reasonable expectation would be one to three complex tasks a week. This is what I found worked for me.

Now look at your list of want-to-do items. Select one or two items. These are items you will reward yourself with after you have completed each task. You and your brain need fun too. So don't forget to plan fun or relaxation time in your day. Otherwise, your brain will let you forget to take time to relax and rest.

Use a timer to remind you to stop your rest break or fun time so you

---

[54] Babauta, *Zen to Done*.

don't forget to go back to work on your next task for the day.

Planning Your Day

Ideally you should create your daily to-do list the evening before the next day. This way you can wake up and start your day with working first on the most complex tasks when your energy is highest.

Plan your daily goal list from your main to-do list and your calendar. Write the day's planned task either in your small notebook you keep in your pocket or in your recovery journal under the day's journal entry. Use your calendar along with your main to-do list when selecting items to help prioritize tasks based on when they need to get done.

You should use a calendar that is a month at a glance. A weekly calendar limits your thinking and planning to one week at a time. When you have a head injury, you need more time to plan and prep for events. In her book, *Mild Traumatic Brain Injury: The Guidebook*, Mary Lou Acimovic says, "An injured brain doesn't do as well at previewing upcoming events."[55] You may need to reference your calendar multiple times a day to help you stay on track.

It's best to use an 8" × 11" calendar. This size will help prevent your calendar from getting lost in your bag or on a cluttered counter. It should have large boxes for each day that will allow you to write appointment times, bill due dates, and other memory-cue notes.

When I'm home on my days off, I write my daily to-do list in a small notebook I keep in my pocket as I move around the house. When at work, I write my daily to-do list on my printed patient schedule. By keeping my list close to me, it reminds me of what I need to do and keeps my focus on the day's planned tasks. I also glance at my daily to-do list for support when I feel overwhelmed and frozen.

---

[55] Acimovic, *Mild Traumatic Brain Injury*, 173.

When you're done for the day, review your list. Move your uncompleted items to the top of your daily to-do list for the next day. If you have room for additional tasks, review your main list along with your calendar and select an item that needs to be done.

How to Create Your Daily To-Do List

Use your calendar to see when items are due when selecting the next day's daily to-do list items from your main to-do list. Write items in your daily pocketbook or a piece of paper you will keep on your desk.

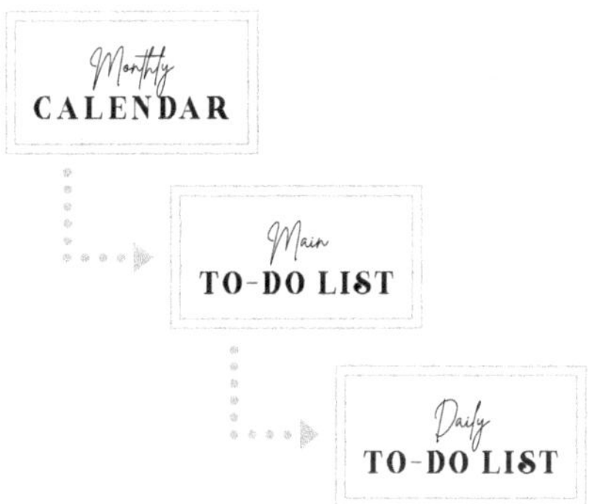

As you accomplish your tasks and goals, mark them as done on your main list.

To help with your motivation, set a timer and commit to working on a task for 15 to 20 minutes. Eliminate all other distractions to prevent your attention or focus from being pulled away during the time you are working on this task. Turn off phones, notification alerts, music, and the TV.

When your timer goes off, rest and take a break.

If you start to feel tired, irritable, or frustrated, stop working on your to-do list. This is your brain telling you that you need to rest. The items you did not get done can then be moved to the next day's list of tasks.

Random, but Important Stuff

As I said before, when your routine is changed, your memory will most likely fail you. In her book, *Mild Traumatic Brain Injury: The Guidebook*, Mary Lou Acimovic recommends "for these times to use sticky notes, to pull your brain's memory additional attention to this new thing you want to remember."[56]

You can use these sticky notes when you need to stop at the grocery store or gas station before driving home. If you need to drop something off at the post office, have the item or letters set right beside you as a reminder to stop at the post office. Remember, out of sight, out of mind.

This has worked for me. For example, I like to have soy milk with my coffee at work. When my box of soy milk runs low at work, I make a sticky note to remind myself to pack a box into my work bag when I get home. I place this note on the outside of my calendar. When I get home and pull my calendar out to plan the next day, the note is there. This is important to me. Without it, I can't enjoy my coffee at work.

Recap

1. Use to-do lists to shift your mental load from your brain onto paper.
2. To-do lists will help you stay organized and focused while your brain heals.
3. Do not expect to manage a to-do list early in your recovery. Managing a to-do list is a complex task.
4. A good indicator you're ready to start managing a to-do list is when you feel comfortable completing your routine daily checkoff lists.
5. You should practice managing to-do lists prior to returning to work and school.
6. To prevent losing track of your main to-do list, keep it in your recovery journal.

---

[56] Acimovic, *Mild Traumatic Brain Injury*, 33.

7. Create your daily to-do lists the evening before from your main to-do list and your calendar.

Chapter 17

Learning How to Learn Again

AFTER YOUR HEAD INJURY, you may feel stupid and slow. You might even believe you will never learn anything new again. If this sounds like you, don't fall prey to negative self-talk.

First, you're not stupid, so tell those negative Nancy, self-doubting voices in your head to shut up. Amanda Rabinowitz and Harvey Levin write in their article, "Cognitive Sequelae of Traumatic Brain Injury," that "TBI patients generally retain the ability to recognize newly learned material."[57] After a head injury, most people's abilities to learn and retain new information are not broken.

But a head injury can affect the way you process and learn new things. As your brain heals, it has limited energy to support the complicated task of comprehending, analyzing, storing, and retaining new information in your memory. Also, its processing function has been wacked off-line with

---

[57] Amanda Rabinowitz and Harvey S. Levin, "Cognitive Sequelae of Traumatic Brain Injury," *The Psychiatric Clinics of North America* 37, no. 1 (March 2014): 3, https://www.doi.org/10.1016/j.psc.2013.11.004.

delays, slowdowns, and backfires. But don't despair. Once you understand what's going on with your brain, the better you will understand new ways of learning.

SLOTH MODE

Learning requires a well-functioning memory. Both brain functions are complex, and there are books devoted to how the brain learns and how memories are formed and retained.

After a head injury, your memory is still intact. The issue is not a shortage of memory space. Amanda Rabinowitz and Harvey Levin in their article, "Cognitive Sequelae of Traumatic Brain Injury," further explain that "TBI patients tend to have difficulties organizing new information for successful encoding and retrieval."[58] Your brain is attempting to take in the information at its normal speed. However, after a head injury your brain's processing speed has slowed down—even if it's only a couple hundredths of a second. Though this delay between the uptake of information and processing the information is minuscule, it's enough to throw a wrench into your cognitive works.

This is the same delay when it comes to your brain's ability to retrieve information and bring it to the forefront of your mind. This delay is finite, but you'll feel as if you're thinking in sloth mode.

This misaligned timing in the brain's information process leads to storage mishaps that can cause delays in retrieval of the new information. This slow processing can even sometimes shut down your brain as it gets overwhelmed.

Think of a conveyor belt carrying boxes of information into a storage room where one sloth oversees filing the information as it comes in and another sloth is responsible for pulling files to be delivered to the front desk. Picture it: Papers fly everywhere, and boxes pile up, making a mess on the

---

[58] Rabinowitz and Levin, "Cognitive Sequelae," 5.

floor, as your sloth diligently files one piece of learned information at a time. That's your brain, and unfortunately, for now it's a sloth.

You're Not Stupid

Understand that you're not stupid. You don't need to smash your laptop or punch your hand through a wall. Stop and take a deep breath. Think about how you learned in the past. What is not working now, and what strategies are in the chapters of this book? Which ones do you need to support your brain's learning process as your brain heals?

Start by using strategies that slow the rate of the incoming information. Decreasing your reading speed and taking information in small doses, for example, can help. Take time to think about what you read, thereby allowing your brain to process the information and file it correctly. This means you will need more time to learn. This is another accommodation you should consider requesting from your instructors, trainers, and employers.

Repetition is also a helpful learning technique. Repeat what you have read or listened to, and solidify the new information you're trying to learn. Writing new information down on notes or note cards to review later is another useful technique.

Once you know what works best through trial and error, you'll be able to start learning by using your brain and external supportive strategies. Remember to be kind to yourself. Challenge your brain, but don't push it to the point of developing headaches, fatigue, dizziness, or irritability.

Your Brain Still Works—It Just Needs Crutches

If you broke your leg, you wouldn't expect your injured leg to help you walk. You wouldn't tell yourself to "just shake it off." You would rest so your leg could heal, use crutches to walk, and complete rehab to slowly build back its strength.

Your brain needs that same care. Don't expect your brain to learn early in your recovery. Give your brain time to heal and expand its energy stamina. Then start to seek new ways to learn that work best for you and your brain.

A Change in Learning Styles

Step one is discovering your new learning style. Dr. Gail Denton, author of *Brainlash: Maximize Your Recovery from Mild Brain Injury,* says, "You need to know as much about your learning style as possible so that you can continue to succeed in your daily life."[59]

Learning styles can be either or a combination of visual, auditory, reading and writing, or sensory. A sensory learner is a kinesthetic learner who learns best from hands-on learning. Before my head injury, I learned best from reading and writing first, then seeing a demonstration of the new information. From there I was ready for hands-on learning.

After my head injury, I was bummed out to find out that I could not read for hours on end anymore. It was a devastating blow to find I could only read for 10 minutes at most. When I did read, I often forgot what I'd just read.

I realized I could not rely on reading as my only avenue for learning. As reading is a complicated task for the brain and a process that consumes a lot of brain energy, I knew I had to adapt to this new situation. Before my head injury, I was not an auditory learner. I learned best from printed words. After my head injury, I was surprised to discover that I could learn by listening to audiobooks.

While your brain heals, consider listening to books to see if you are now an auditory learner. You may find you retain information better when listening as compared to reading.

---

[59] Denton, *Brainlash*, 83.

You can also purchase the hard text of a book. This will enable you to use the text as a reference to help you recall information you may have learned but forgotten. Then when you want to reread or reference the information again, you'll have that information printed on eye- and brain-friendly paper.

Instructional videos are also excellent learning tools. This way the brain is learning from listening to the audio at the same time your eyes follow the words or graphic demonstrations on the video. You can further support your brain filing this new information by taking notes. As you watch the video, hit pause while you write down the information in your notes. I found that watching a video helped reinforce my learning with less brain drain. Thanks, YouTube!

Learning from videos, audio recordings, prerecorded presentations, and lectures gives you the benefit of being able to rewind or replay when you need to review information. This is a great way to capture information when you're not understanding what's being said or your attention wanders off while the video is playing. You can also hit pause to stop and write down notes you can reference later. Also ask your instructors and managers to provide training and instructions in writing. This allows you to review what was discussed at your own pace.

Consider asking if your instructors will let you record their lectures. This will allow you to relisten to the presented information at your brain's processing speed. Many audio apps and computers let you select the speed at which the text is read, allowing you to slow down the information to match your brain's processing speed.

Speech Therapy and Neuropsychology

If you're having problems with learning or memory processes, see a speech therapist. Speech therapy is not all about helping people articulate their words better. Speech therapists are amazing health care professionals who can help you reestablish learning and memory following a head injury. They can provide great insight to help you discover where the hang-up is in your learning process and provide you with strategies and exercises to help you with your memory and learning process.

Another resource is seeing a neuropsychologist. These health care professionals can perform a neuropsychological evaluation. This test identifies areas in your brain's cognitive function that aren't working well. This test is extensive (taking an entire day to complete) and expensive. I completed this test, and it helped me understand why I felt as if I was barely keeping my head above the water with work and life. It also reassured me that I had not lost too many IQ points after my head injury.

Trying harder to learn does not work with a healing brain. Your brain, in time, will reward you with better comprehension, retention, and retrieval of new information.

RECAP

1. Learn how your brain likes to learn.
2. Try finding alternatives to reading, like audiobooks.
3. Experiment with instructional videos and audio instructions.
4. Support your learning with external memory tools, and reinforce learning techniques.
5. Be patient, take a deep breath, and slow your information intake down.

Section IV

Lifestyle

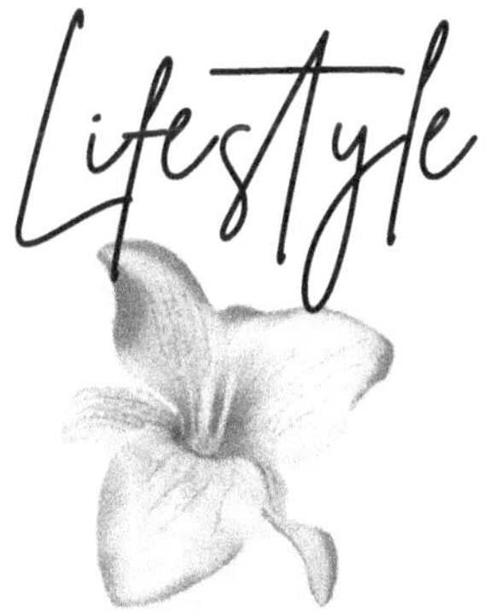

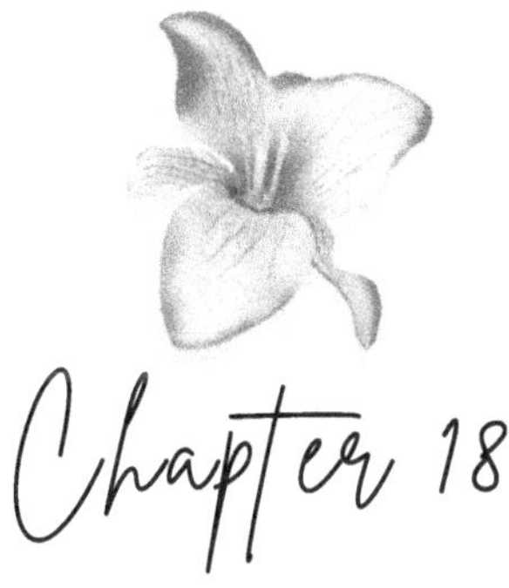

Chapter 18
Lifestyle
Live Long and Prosper

SUSTAINING A HEAD INJURY unfortunately puts you at risk of developing neurodegenerative diseases, such as Alzheimer's as well as some forms of dementia. I remember reading this while I was recovering from my head injury and thinking sarcastically, "Great, that's exactly what I want to hear." Later in my recovery, I learned what I could do to lower my risk of dementia.

High-quality sleep, exercise, mindful thinking, and brain-healthy nutrition are all keys to your recovery and maintaining the integrity of your cognitive function going forward. It will be essential for you to embrace this lifestyle to help you recover from your head injury.

FOUNDATION FOR RECOVERY AND THE FUTURE

- **Sleep:** Sleep is the foundation of recovery. When you go to sleep, your brain goes into high gear to clean out toxins, repair damage, organize your memories, and address your emotional stress.

- **Exercise:** It's common after a head injury to lack energy and motivation to exercise. You may even find yourself becoming surprisingly winded even after minimal effort. This is why it's important to start slow, be safe, and stay persistent in your efforts because exercise will help rejuvenate your mind and body. Exercise also prevents brain atrophy (shrinkage), which can increase your risk of developing dementia later in life.

- **Mindfulness:** After a head injury, it's easy to get lost in your own mind and feel as if you're sharing your body with a stranger. Mindfulness will help you get out of your head and away from the whirling thoughts of stress and worry. It will clarify and help you reexamine your passions and core values, which sometimes change after a head injury. It will also help you get to know your brain and discover the new you.

- **Nutrition:** The cellular damage from a brain injury can ignite a biochemical cascade that can affect your brain's functions. The last thing your brain needs is poor nutrition full of fat, sugar, salt, and toxins when it is trying to heal. Eating a brain-healthy diet will be the weapon you wield to fight for your recovery and shield your brain against the detrimental effects of chronic illnesses that can increase your risk of Alzheimer's and vascular dementia.

- **Livelihood:** A head injury can affect your financial security. It's hard to be motivated to embrace a healthy lifestyle when you're stressed about paying your bills.

The truth is, getting better and staying healthy are up to you. I believe these lifestyle behaviors are what helped me recover and grow stronger after my head injury. I hope you take this ball of information and run with it happily through your recovery and into the future.

Chapter 19

Sleep Is the Foundation of Recovery

SLEEP IS AN IMPORTANT function of the brain. Sleep is like having a personal trainer, an efficient office manager, a certified psychologist, and a janitor all wrapped up in one neat little package. While you sleep, your brain sorts and files all your memories from the previous day. It finds the strength to manage your emotions and recharge your prefrontal cortex. This helps you maintain rational thinking and decision-making and puts the brakes on strong emotions such as rage and anger. While you sleep, researchers have noted that your brain works to improve your motor skills, lower your blood pressure, control your blood sugar, combat obesity, and support a robust immune system.[60] Sleep is also responsible for cleaning out cellular waste products that can build up inside your brain and cause severe health problems. If you get less than six hours of sleep at night, you have an increased risk of stroke and developing cancer, and Alzheimer's dementia. As you age, you don't want to add these health issues on top of a head injury.

---

[60] Walker, *Why We Sleep,* 170–71.

What Is Quality Sleep?

It's imperative during recovery that you get high-quality sleep in order to care properly for your brain. A normal sleep pattern starts with falling asleep within 20 minutes of laying down. A normal sleep pattern includes waking up once or twice during the night and being able to resume sleeping within 20 minutes.

Sleep researchers recommend that everyone should get seven to nine hours of sleep at night. Dr. Cheryle Sullivan in her book, *Brain Injury Survival Kit*, said, "People who have had brain injuries often need even more sleep than those without brain injuries, as much as 10+ hours a night."[61] Emerson Wickwire and colleagues reported, "Patients with TBI slept two-and-a-half hours longer per 24-hour period."[62] Therefore, it's normal to expect that after your head injury you will be sleeping more hours than you did prior to your head injury.

In his book, *Why We Sleep*, Matthew Walker shares that "insufficient sleep appears to be a key lifestyle factor linked to your risk of developing Alzheimer's disease."[63] This may explain why it is suggested that people who sleep six hours or less at night are at a higher risk of developing Alzheimer's dementia.

Sleep Is a Complex Brain Process

If you're having trouble getting seven to nine hours of sleep at night, see your general health care provider for help. There are some common sleep disorders that may disrupt your sleep after having a head injury.

---

[61] Sullivan, *Brain Injury Survival Kit*, 11.

[62] Emerson Wickwire et al., "Sleep, Sleep Disorders and Mild Traumatic Brain Injury. What We Know and What We Need to Know: Findings from a National Working Group," *Neurotherapeutics* 13, no. 2 (April 2016): 409, https://www.doi.org/10.1007/s13311-016-0429-3.

[63] Walker, *Why We Sleep*, 3.

Following a head injury, certain sleep processes in your brain may be knocked off-line, such as your circadian rhythm, which tells us when to be awake or asleep. Emerson Wickwire explains, "It is clear that sleep disturbances and resultant sleep disorders can impair the brain injury recovery process."[64]

Sleep involves brain structures, neurotransmitters, and hormones—all of which can be damaged or disrupted by a head injury. This can leave you with a sleep disorder such as insomnia, fragmented sleep, or obstructive sleep apnea.

Insomnia is when you're not able to fall asleep or when your sleep is fragmented, causing you to wake up for an hour or two at night or very early in the morning. The first three months after my head injury, I had both insomnia and fragmented sleep.

At first, I had a hard time going to sleep because of my fear of having a car-related nightmare. Later on, I developed fragmented sleep, waking up at three a.m. and being unable to fall back asleep for a couple hours. On occasion I would wake up one hour before my alarm went off and could not go back to sleep. This created anxiety because I knew the next day would be a miserable brain day.

Obstructive sleep apnea (OSA) is when you stop breathing while you are sleeping. I have patients who don't know that they have this sleep disorder, though they will report issues with daytime sleepiness, fatigue, and falling asleep when sitting down to watch a movie or the TV. Emerson Wickwire explains, "Obstructive sleep apnea occurs at a substantially higher rate in patients with TBI than the general population."[65] He further explains that patients with brain injuries and untreated OSA will have increased difficulty with attention and memory.[66] In general, untreated OSA has been found to increase your risk of heart attack, stroke, cancer, and dementia.

---

[64] Wickwire et al., "Sleep, Sleep Disorders," 404.
[65] Wickwire et al., "Sleep, Sleep Disorders," 410.
[66] Wickwire et al., "Sleep, Sleep Disorders," 410.

Your health care provider can refer you to be screened for OSA. This testing requires you to wear a device on your hand and a small strip around your chest while you are sleeping at home. Once the test is completed, it's analyzed by a sleep doctor who will make treatment recommendations based on your test results.

Learn How to Sleep

So, if you've suffered a head injury and are having trouble sleeping, how do you get the high-quality sleep that you need to recover? First you must allow sufficient time to get at least seven to nine hours of sleep a night. To get started, first calculate what Matthew Walker terms as your "sleep opportunity window."[67]

This is the time frame that will help you get the minimum of seven to nine hours of sleep. So, I need an average of nine hours of sleep per night. Therefore, I have a 10-hour sleep opportunity window. I must be up for work by 7:30 a.m. and need to go to sleep at 9:30 p.m. to fulfill this requirement. My sleep opportunity window then is between 9:30 p.m. and 7:30 a.m.

The other important thing to institute is a sleep hygiene routine, which is a routine you do two hours prior to bedtime. Sleep is a learned behavior, and a pre-bedtime routine can help start the brain's sleep function. It has also been shown to be more effective with helping most people sleep than sleep medications.[68]

A good sleep routine should start with no TV or use of media devices two hours before you want to go to sleep. The lights should be dimmed and sound quieted. Select a relaxing activity of either doing the dishes, picking up the kids' toys, putting away some laundry, reading a book, or listening to relaxing music.

---

[67] Walker, *Why We Sleep*, 291.
[68] Walker, *Why We Sleep*, 291.

One hour before bed, take a shower or bath with relaxing music and candles. Your bedroom should be electronic-free, without TVs or computers. It should also be dark and cool.

Sometimes I have difficulty falling asleep because my mind will not turn off. I found listening to a book or sleep music helps distract me from these whirling thoughts. I've also found that writing down things I want to remember in my pocket journal I keep at the bedside at night helps me let go of thoughts I want to remember for the next day.

I recommend that you keep track of the hours you sleep and the quality of your sleep. This will let you know if you're short on sleep and need to make up for it the next night.[69] Plus, you can plan your day based on the quality of sleep you have been getting. When I know I have not slept well, I plan to get just the minimum done the next day.

I use a Fitbit to track my sleep. My Fitbit tells me the hours I sleep, if I was restless, how many times I woke up in the night, and how long it took me to fall back to sleep. It also calculates the percentage of my sleep spent in wakefulness, REM, deep sleep, and light sleep. I advise you to consider investing in a device that monitors sleep for yourself.

WHEN YOUR SLEEP IS BROKEN

It's common for my patients with head injuries or neurologic issues to struggle with sleep. Emerson Wickwire says, "Head injuries may affect normal melatonin production."[70]

I often recommend to my patients to take melatonin every night as a first-line treatment for insomnia. I've found it helps my patients fall asleep and also smooths out fragmented sleep patterns.

Melatonin is a hormone released by the brain as the day's light grows

---

[69] Shingo Kitamura et al., "Estimating Individual Optimal Sleep Duration and Potential Sleep Debt," *Scientific Reports* 6, no. 35812 (2016): 5, https://doi.org/10.1038/srep35812.
[70] Wickwire et al., "Sleep, Sleep Disorders," 410.

darker. The light from smart devices can decrease melatonin levels by 20%. Mathew Walker shares, "Compared to reading a printed book, reading on an iPad suppressed melatonin release by over 50%."[71] This is why it is important to avoid bright lights, the TV, and media devices two hours prior to you wanting to fall asleep.

For my patients who are 69 years or younger, I generally recommend starting out with five milligrams a half hour prior to wanting to fall asleep. If my patients are 70 years or older, I recommend they start out with three milligrams of melatonin a half hour prior to bedtime. I also advise that they take this dose for a minimum of two months to see the full effectiveness. This is because melatonin is a supplement. It also is not habit forming, unlike some sleeping medications. If needed, I adjust the dose and timing of it every two months. If you find you are taking 10 milligrams of melatonin at night, and it's not improving your sleep, consult with your general practitioner before increasing the dose.

RECAP

1. It's recommended that you get seven to nine hours of sleep every night, but after a head injury, you may need even more.
2. See your general practitioner if you develop insomnia or fragmented sleep.
3. Take sleep apnea seriously and be 100% compliant with the recommended treatment.
4. Sleep is a learned behavior supported by good sleep hygiene and a nightly routine.
5. Read or listen to Matthew Walker's book, *Why We Sleep*, on Audible.com for more information on sleep.

---

[71] Walker, *Why We Sleep*, 269–70.

Chapter 20

Mindfulness

RECOVERING FROM A HEAD injury can be a long and lonely process. Recovery will hinge on the ability to rediscover yourself and let go of what was lost because of your head injury. If you stay in your head with negative thoughts, replaying past events, and worrying about what-ifs, your recovery may hit a dead end. This could cause you to spend your life beating your fists against an unyielding wall in the company of anxiety, depression, and exhaustion.

Mindfulness, journaling, and mental health therapy will get you out of your head so you can be present in the world around you. These strategies can help you realize that it's possible to walk around the wall instead of trying to go through it.

WHAT IS MINDFUL THINKING

Practicing mindfulness means living in the moment. It's a practice that pulls your thoughts away from your past regrets and future worries and places your awareness on the now.

Christopher Bergland further explains that "mindfulness is simply about being mindful of what you're thinking and deciding where you choose to focus your attention."[72] It gets you out of your mental rut and brings your awareness to the present.

Mindfulness Is a Great Tool for Your Toolbox

The practice of mindfulness is a great tool to use while you're recovering from your head injury. Dr. Eva Hvingelby says in her article, "Mindfulness Supports Healing After Head Trauma," that mindfulness "can help relieve pain, improve sleep and increase hopefulness about the future."[73] Rebecca L. Acabchuk says that there is now promising evidence that meditation, yoga, and mindfulness-based interventions can lead to modest improvements in symptoms of head trauma, particularly in fatigue, depression, and quality of life.[74] These benefits in turn will help you to continue to work and study while your brain is healing.

Mindfulness has also shown to help with controlling your emotions and improving your communication with others during stressful situations. Mindfulness practice has helped me sit calmly while sitting through stressful work meetings. When you practice mindfulness, it allows you and your brain a moment to analyze your feelings toward stressful situations

---

[72] Christopher Bergland, "Mindfulness Made Simple," *The Athlete's Way* (blog), *Psychology Today*, March 31, 2013, https://www.psychologytoday.com/us/blog/the-athletes-way/201303/mindfulness-made-simple.

[73] Eva Hvingelby, "Mindfulness Supports Healing After Head Trauma," Verywell Health, modified January 15, 2020, https://www.verywellhealth.com/mindfulness-supports-healing-after-head-trauma-4059399.

[74] Jaclyn Severance, "First Meta-Analysis Shows Promise for Yoga, Meditation, Mindfulness in Concussion," Science Daily, November 30, 2020, https://www.sciencedaily.com/releases/2020/11/201130131439.htm; R, L. Acabchuk, J. M. Brisson, C. L. Park, N. Babbott-Bryan, O. A. Parmelee, B. T. Johnson. *Therapeutic Effects of Meditation, Yoga, and Mindfulness-Based Interventions for Chronic Symptoms of Mild Traumatic Brain Injury: A Systematic Review and Meta-Analysis.* Appl Psychol Health Well Being. 2021 Feb;13(1):34-62. doi: 10.1111/aphw.12244. Epub 2020 Nov 2. PMID: 33136346. https://pubmed.ncbi.nlm.nih.gov/33136346/

and then respond in an appropriate way. This is key when maintaining your interpersonal and professional relationships at home, school, or work.

You may be thinking that mindfulness sounds weird or complicated. If you decide to try it out, you may wonder if you're doing it right or think you need to invest more time. Christopher Bergland points out that "you don't have to set aside time to sit quietly in the lotus position and burn incense to practice mindfulness. You can do it anytime, anywhere."[75]

While you might be thinking to yourself, "There's no way I can sit, meditate, and stay awake at the same time." You may believe you just don't have time to try and practice mindfulness between work and taking care of your family.

These are some legitimate concerns but practicing mindful thinking doesn't have to be complicated. You can practice it anywhere, and it only takes one to two minutes. (Eventually you can lengthen your practice time.) It's also possible to practice while you're cooking, talking with a loved one, or sitting at work or out on your deck at home.

For example, while you're cooking, take a moment to enjoy the vibrant colors of your vegetables as you slice them up for your meal. For just a minute, focus your attention on how the knife feels in your hand as it chops up your vegetables. Then take a little time to run your fingers through a bowl of beans and feel their textures as you rinse them under the water.

Mindfulness can be practiced when you're talking to your loved ones. To do so, put down your smart devices and turn off the TV. Then sit and take a few deep breaths as you listen to what they're saying and the sound of their voice. As you're listening, focus on their facial and hand expressions. Keep your mind clear and don't allow your brain to think about what you want to say or what you need to get done after the conversation. Instead, encourage your brain to focus only on the moment and the conversation.

At work, whenever you have time, practice by closing your eyes and

---

[75] Bergland, "Mindfulness Made Simple."

taking a minute to focus on taking five deep breaths. Sometimes when I'm at my desk, I'll grab a mini coloring book and color in a small flower or ladybug for a quick calming mental reprieve.

My favorite time to practice mindfulness is at home while sitting on my deck. I sit and take intermittent deep breaths, noting the surrounding smells, the changing colors of the sky as the sun sets, and the sounds of neighborhood kids playing, people talking, and dogs barking. I watch squirrels and birds flit through the trees over my head.

There are also smartphone apps that can guide you through mindful moments. I recommend starting out by spending time coloring in adult coloring books. I found focusing on coloring opened my mind to how mindfulness works and feels, which I used as a guide to try and practice other mindfulness techniques.

How to Get Started

At first you may need to start slow, setting aside one to two minutes a day to practice and build the length of your sessions from there. By doing this, you'll make practicing mindfulness a priority for your brain. It's perfectly fine to schedule your mindfulness into your daily routine, just as you do with exercise. When I started, I had to use an alarm on my smartphone to remind me to take a moment to practice my mindful thinking.

Puzzles and Coloring

Early in your recovery you may have little energy for physical activities, and you might be more interested in beginning with mindful practices you can do sitting down. These can include working on craft projects or sitting quietly outside.

You can also practice mindful thinking while drawing, coloring, working on a do-it-yourself project, putting a puzzle together, or while knitting. The key is to be focused in the moment and tune into your body and breathing.

Start your mindfulness practice by choosing what you're going to focus on. Turn off any other distractions such as your smart devices, TV, and music. While you're focused on your project, take deep breaths intermittently while noticing the feel of your lungs filling with air and chest deflating as you exhale. As you're working on your chosen project, focus your attention on the colors and textures of the material you're working with and how they feel in your hands.

For example, if you're putting a puzzle together, observe closely the color of each puzzle piece and how the light hits and reflects off the completed part of the puzzle. Pay attention to how each puzzle piece you select feels between your fingers as it snaps into place.

I love to knit while sitting on the couch in front of a roaring fire. As I knit, my attention goes to my breathing as I appreciate the color and feel of the yarn and my knitting needles as I work on making my stitches. I listen to the quiet roar and sparks from the fire as I interweave my yarn. I think of the people I'm knitting my scarf or hat for and how grateful I am that they're in my life.

These moments in the here and now will help you learn how mindfulness feels. The more you practice, the better your brain will perform when dealing with mental stress or distractions.

WALKING AND YOGA

When your physical injuries have healed and you're feeling stronger, you can start incorporating active mindfulness into your recovery. Two practices that I recommend to my patients are walking and yoga.

Mindful walking outdoors offers several benefits for your brain and body. Dr. Eva Hvingelby writes, "During mindful walking, several things are happening. You are maintaining an awareness of the breath in your body. You are also paying particular attention to coordination, balance, the feel of the ground under your feet and the air on your skin. The brain is slowing its thoughts to remain in the present moment and see, hear, feel, everything."[76] She further explains that this helps retrain your brain to pay attention to the important information it is sensing in your environment and to stay focused in the moment.[77]

Yoga is another excellent option I recommend to my patients because it helps build strength, improve flexibility, and tone core muscles, which helps heal neck and back injuries that may have been sustained along with your head injury. Yoga practice will also bring awareness to your posture and balance, which will help decrease symptoms of dizziness and risk of falls.

Yoga teaches you breathing techniques and boosts your mental and physical awareness to help with your mindfulness practice. Yoga has been found by researchers to help the brain cells create new connections that can improve cognitive function, memory, attention, and learning skills after a head injury.[78]

Researchers reported that brain imaging scans of people who practiced yoga regularly showed less brain atrophy then those who did not practice yoga.[79] Yoga not only will gently heal your body, but the practice of mindfulness while you are doing yoga helps heal your brain.

The good news is, you can learn yoga from a class, online videos, or a smart device app. I took a beginning yoga class that was a series of two classes a week for four weeks. I learned a lot and was able to continue practicing my yoga at home. If you decide you would like to attend class at a yoga studio, let the instructors know about any injuries, balance difficulties,

---

76 Hvingelby, "Mindfulness Supports Healing."

77 Hvingelby, "Mindfulness Supports Healing."

78 Ling Beisecker, "This Is How Yoga Benefits Your Brain," Do You, modified August 5, 2016, https://www.doyou.com/this-is-how-yoga-benefits-your-brain-1797802-47478/.

79 Brett Froeliger, Eric L. Garland, and F. Joseph McClernon, "Yoga Meditation Practitioners Exhibit Greater Gray Matter Volume and Fewer Reported Cognitive Failures: Results of a Preliminary Voxel-Based Morphometric Analysis," *Evidence-Based Complementary and Alternative Medicine* 2012 (December 2012): 6, https://www.doi.org/10.1155/2012/821307.

or memory issues. Your instructor can help modify your yoga practice to best accommodate your needs. That's one of the many great things about yoga—there's more than one way to practice.

You will see the full effectiveness of your mindful thinking when you practice with intent on a regular basis.[80] If you struggle with your mindfulness practice, seek support from your counselor or psychologist. As you practice your mindfulness over time, you'll get better at it and begin to reap all of the rewards it has to offer.

Get Out of Your Head

Other ways you might practice mindful thinking are knitting, gardening, and organizing drawers and cabinets in your home. You can also learn from your mental health providers other ways to practice mindfulness, like meditation, deep breathing exercises, and ways to be more in the moment.

My counselor introduced me to practicing mindfulness with coloring in adult coloring books. Dr. Eva Hvingelby said, "There are numerous studies that support music and art therapy as successful in helping a traumatized brain recover from its injuries. Similar to mindfulness training, being immersed in beautiful sounds or focusing on drawing or sculpting puts worrisome thoughts that contribute to stress and fear into the background."[81] Early into my recovery, my coloring helped me get out of my head that was too often cluttered with worry and stressful thoughts.

I've grown to love adult coloring during the years of my recovery. I find it relaxing, and the act of coloring helps focus my mind and thoughts into the present moment.

---

[80] Alicia Nortje, "How to Practice Mindfulness: 11 Practical Steps and Tips," Positive Psychology, March 23, 2022, https://positivepsychology.com/how-to-practice-mindfulness/.

[81] Hvingelby, "Mindfulness Supports Healing."

RECAP

Practicing mindfulness can help you in the following ways:

1. Let go of what you lost due to your head injury.
2. Bring to focus your new passions and core values.
3. Reduce mental stress and improve your focus.
4. Allow you to get to know your brain and the new you.

I hope you consider trying mindful thinking. I've found it to be one of the best tools I've accessed during my recovery, and it helps me to move forward with caring for myself and my brain. It's also a great way to give your brain a break and bring clarity of thought to your mind. I will warn you though—if you start adult coloring or knitting like me, you may develop an addiction to coloring pencils, adult coloring books, and yarn.

Chapter 21

Exercise

I WAS SHOCKED TO find that when I started exercising two weeks after my head injury, I went from being able to do two hours of martial arts training to being winded after a couple minutes. I mistakenly continued to push through exhaustion, which worsened my injury.

Kurt Mossberg says, "A sedentary lifestyle and lack of endurance are common characteristics of individuals with TBI who have a reduction in peak aerobic capacity of 25% to 30% compared to healthy sedentary persons."[82] To this day, I can't keep up with my 70-year-old dad when we go hiking. He just laughs at me as he leaves me huffing and puffing in the dust.

Scientists have not been able to explain the exact mechanism as to why after a head injury there is a noted reduction in your cardio fitness. In their article, "Improving Cardiorespiratory Fitness with Aerobic Exercise Training in Individuals with Traumatic Brain Injury," Lisa Chin

---

[82] Kurt A. Mossberg, William E. Amonette, and Brent E. Masel, "Endurance Training and Cardiorespiratory Conditioning After Traumatic Brain Injury," *The Journal of Head Trauma Rehabilitation* 25, no. 3 (May–June 2010): 173, https://www.doi.org/10.1097/HTR.0b013e3181dc98ff.

and colleagues believe some factors could be due to deconditioning of your body after prolonged rest during your early recovery.[83]

SAFETY FIRST

Early into recovery, you shouldn't push yourself physically to the point of being exhausted or in pain. It will be important for you to move and be active, but the exercise needs to be within your limits and safe.

It's best to be active most days of the week. Keep in mind you don't have to go to the gym to exercise. There are plenty of activities to choose from, and it's best to pick one that you enjoy and find rewarding.

I often tell my patients that exercise should be rejuvenating to the body and mind and have a relaxing effect on your muscles. If you're exhausted and have discomfort after exercising, then you know you have pushed yourself too hard.

I recommend avoiding high-impact sports and activities that increase your risk for head injuries, such as snowboarding, skiing, and mountain biking. Personally, another head injury just isn't worth it, knowing that head injuries are cumulative. Each time you hit your head it will take longer for you to recover. For this reason, I gave up snowboarding and downhill skiing.

You should avoid activities that require rapid response times. After a head injury, it's common to move slowly, feel off-balance, and have a slower reaction time. So, you may want to skip playing sports like tennis, basketball, fencing, or dodge ball until your reaction time is back up to speed.

Instead, consider walking, swimming, dancing, Pilates, yoga, hiking, or gardening. I believe the best exercises to start with after a head injury are walking and gentle yoga. Whichever exercise you choose, get moving

---

[83] Lisa M. K. Chin et al., "Improving Cardiorespiratory Fitness with Aerobic Exercise Training in Individuals with Traumatic Brain Injury," *The Journal of Head Trauma Rehabilitation* 30, no. 6 (November–December 2015): 389.

and help your body and your brain cells stay healthy. Pick an exercise or several different exercises you enjoy doing throughout the week. Get active and be safe.

WHY EXERCISE?

Exercise has been shown in people with brain injuries to improve mood, creativity, decrease stress, lower stress hormones, and help with pain control. My patients tell me often how exercise also helps them sleep better at night.

Staying active will be an important component to your recovery process and maintaining your brain health for the future. According to Romain Meeusen, "Exercise has been promoted as a possible prevention for neurodegenerative disease."[84] This means every time you go for a walk, you're lowering your risk for developing dementia.

If you don't exercise, you may develop additional chronic diseases that increase your risk for stroke, dementia, or diabetes. There is some research that suggest that exercise helps lower fatigue in patients with traumatic brain injuries.[85] Other researchers believe that physically active traumatic brain injury survivors have a higher likelihood of returning to work and school, compared to TBI survivors who are sedentary.[86]

START SLOW AND GENTLE

When beginning an exercise routine, start out slow. The activity you choose

---

[84] Romain Meeusen, "Exercise, Nutrition and the Brain," *Sports Medicine* 44, no. 1 (May 2014): 47, https://www.doi.org/10.1007/s40279-014-0150-5.

[85] Chin et al., "Improving Cardiorespiratory Fitness," 382.

[86] Timothy P. Morris et al., "Traumatic Brain Injury Modifies the Relationship Between Physical Activity and Global and Cognitive Health: Results from the Barcelona Brain Health Initiative," *Frontiers in Behavioral Neuroscience* 13, no. 135 (2019): 2, https://doi.org/10.3389/fnbeh.2019.00135.

needs to be gentle, like walking outside for 10 minutes a day. For example, you can plan to walk five minutes out your door and five minutes back, one to two days a week. Over time, slowly increase your walking time and frequency per week. If you need to take a nap after you exercise, you should cut down on the intensity and length until you feel refreshed from it.

Pay attention to your limits, and pace yourself accordingly. The overall goal after you're feeling stronger is to walk most days of the week for 30 minutes to an hour. Just remember, it's up to you to find a balance between exercising and your daily cognitive energy.

No Time and Too Tired

The most common excuse I get from my patients is not having enough time or energy to exercise. I totally get that. Sometimes just doing physical therapy might wear you out. You might even worry that you'll fall because you feel dizzy or off-balance. These are all valid reasons to not want to exercise.

Early into my recovery, I was barely making it through the work week. During this time, I was significantly less active. When I felt as if I had more energy, my activities were limited to the weekend, which is when I tried to do a little bit of house- and yard work. Three years into my recovery, I started to incorporate more walking and hiking on weekends and on my days off from work. To this day I'm not back to the activity level I was at prior to my head injury. I find that there's not enough energy left over from work to get back to my full workouts. This may be the same for you.

Just do the best you can, exercising when you're strong and resting when you are having a bad brain day. Your goal during your recovery should be to keep your feet wet when it comes to exercise. As your brain heals and your energy levels improve, you will be able to exercise on a more consistent basis.

Getting Motivated

People say it takes discipline to stay fit and exercise. I say first it takes motivation. Previously in this book I talked about lack of motivation following a head injury. I know my motivation fizzles out like a soda pop left open on a hot day when it comes to exercise.

Honestly, I don't like exercising. I would rather cuddle up with a book and my dog on the couch than go out on a walk. It takes a lot to motivate me to exercise, but I know it's good for me, and when it comes down to it, I never regret a workout once I get going, and I often feel refreshed afterward.

When COVID-19 hit the U.S. and I started to work from home, each day was turning into "Blursday" for me. I saw how quickly days would go by with me not exercising. I started to feel my muscles losing strength, and of course I was gaining weight. Here are some recommendations for getting and staying motivated with an easy exercise routine that you won't dread.

1. **Assign yourself workout days:** What can help you get out of a sedentary rut is assigning specific days of the week to exercise. For example, Monday is yoga day for me. That way when I wake up on Monday morning, I know I need to practice yoga.

2. **Set out your workout clothes the night before:** Having my clothes out and ready when I wake helps get me out the door faster for my morning walk.

3. **Plan short exercise sessions:** Sometimes it's easier to get yourself to exercise if you commit to a 15-minute session rather than a half hour. There are also free exercise apps you can download onto your smartphone that will lead you through seven-minute workouts. Starting out with small workouts helps solidify the habit of exercising into your daily routine.

4. **Write down your commitment to exercise on your calendar:** When exercise is scheduled on your calendar, it can motivate and remind you to exercise. This also helps you to see how active you've been and take notice of what you've accomplished.

5. **Consider purchasing a device that counts your steps:** Seeing how many steps I've taken with my Fitbit helps motivate me to go on a walk or get moving more around the house. A similar smart device might help motivate you to get more steps in too.

6. **Consider purchasing walking sticks:** If you have dizziness or feel off balance use recreational walking sticks in each hand while walking or hiking to help you feel more stable and to prevent falls.

7. **Consider chair exercises:** If you don't feel safe with stand-up exercises, consider sitting in a chair or using a chair for balance. There are also videos online (or some you can purchase) that will lead you through various chair workouts. I enjoy doing chair yoga when I'm at work while sitting at my desk and use a chair for balance when I practice my standing yoga poses or martial arts kicks.

8. **Try out yoga:** I recommend yoga to my patients because it enhances muscle strength, aids in flexibility with stretching, improves sleep, and helps manage stress. But not all yoga practices are the same. I recommend restorative, gentle, or chair yoga.

9. **Find a workout partner or group:** If someone is waiting for you, you won't skip your workout.

As the sayings go, "A little bit of something is better than a whole lot of nothing," and "If you don't use it, then you're going to lose it."

RECAP

1. Exercise is important for your brain health, especially after a head injury.
2. You may suffer from fatigue, so it's best to take your exercise slow and easy at first.
3. Create a schedule and a routine that are realistic for you and your healing brain.
4. Every move, yoga pose, and step you take help prevent dementia.
5. Your exercise should leave you and your brain refreshed and rejuvenated.

Chapter 22
The Best Nutrition for Your Brain

DURING YOUR HEAD INJURY, your brain was bounced around inside your skull, stretching and tearing cells while causing a complex cascade of damage. Scientists believe that the damage may linger for months to years after your head injury.[87] Therefore, the food you choose to nourish your brain may be one of the most important aids in your recovery.

After my head injury, it was important for me to protect my cognitive function. I want to live a long, healthy, and active life. However, I was surprised to learn that after a head injury you have a higher risk of developing a neurodegenerative disease such as Alzheimer's.

Dr. Lindsay Wilson and William Stewart et al., in their article, "The Chronic and Evolving Neurological Consequences of Traumatic Brain Injury," state, "TBI represents a risk factor for a variety of neurological

---

[87] Helen M. Bramlett and W. Dalton Dietrich, "Long-Term Consequences of Traumatic Brain Injury: Current Status of Potential Mechanisms of Injury and Neurological Outcomes," *Journal of Neurotrauma* 32, no. 23 (December 2015): 1834, https://www.doi.org/10.1089/neu.2014.3352.

illnesses, including epilepsy, stroke, and neurodegenerative disease."[88]

Eating low-fat, low-toxin, and anti-inflammatory foods for me was imperative. The last thing you want to do is deprive your brain of clean-energy foods. Even healthy brains need nutrition full of antioxidants, fiber, vitamins, minerals, and complex carbohydrates.

In his book, *Power Foods for the Brain: An Effective 3-Step Plan to Protect Your Mind and Strengthen Your Memory*, Dr. Neal D. Barnard says that "specific foods and eating patterns have a powerful protective effect."[89] What I'm recommending is to give your brain the best possible nutrition while it heals and to protect your brain's function from being diminished by disease or vascular malfunction, such as a stroke.

Therefore, I recommend whole-foods, plant-based nutrition. Simply put, it's about eating vegetables and fruits, just as your parents told you when you were a kid.

WHOLE-FOODS, PLANT-BASED NUTRITION

A whole-foods, plant-based diet (WFPB) means choosing to eat more nutrient-dense foods that are close to the soil of a farm and far from a factory. It means deciding to avoid processed foods, which are often high in fat, sugar, and salt. A good example is choosing to eat an orange rather than drink a glass of orange juice. The orange provides you fiber, calcium, potassium, and folate, whereas a glass of orange juice has sugar and preservatives, many times without the good stuff.

A plant-based diet is often lumped into the same category as a vegan diet. However, there are some differences. A WFPB diet avoids processed foods, sugar, salt, fat, and oils, unlike vegan diets, which are focused solely

[88] Lindsay Wilson et al., "The Chronic and Evolving Neurological Consequences of Traumatic Brain Injury," *The Lancet Neurology* 16, no. 10 (October 2017): 813, https://doi.org/10.1016/S1474-4422(17)30279-X.

[89] Neal D. Barnard, *Power Foods for the Brain: An Effective 3-Step Plan to Protect Your Mind and Strengthen Your Memory* (Sanger, CA: Balance, 2014): xvii.

on eliminating animal products and sometimes include low-nutrient, processed foods.

I believe it's important to limit processed foods and animal protein because they usually are high in saturated fat, oil, salt, and sugar. Dr. T. Colin Campbell and Dr. Thomas Campbell II in their book, *The China Study*, found it is best to keep animal protein intake to 10% or less of your total diet.[90]

The reason is that animal products and protein include saturated fat, salt, antibiotics, hormones, and bacteria. In his book *The Healthiest Diet on the Planet,* Dr. John McDougall says, "[Animal products] contain disease-causing microbes (including, but not limited to, mad cow prions; listeria, *E. coli*, and salmonella bacteria; and leukemia viruses) and contain the highest levels of poisonous environmental chemicals found in the food chain."[91] These are the last things you want to feed to your healing brain. Animal protein and dairy are also high in cholesterol, calories, and fat that promote chronic inflammation and do not provide as high of a nutritional value than plant-based foods.

Dr. Joel Fuhrman, in his book *Eat to Live: The Amazing Nutrient-Rich Program for Fast and Sustained Weight Loss,* further explains, Cholesterol levels can be decreased by reducing both saturated fat and animal protein while eating more plant protein.[92]

Diets that include saturated fat and cholesterol can increase your risk of heart attacks, cancer, strokes, and transient ischemic accidents, which are also known as ministrokes that lead over time to vascular dementia. After a head injury, it is imperative to protect your cognitive function from

---

[90] Thomas Campbell and T. Colin Campbell II, *The China Study: The Most Comprehensive Study of Nutrition Ever Conducted and the Startling Implications for Diet, Weight Loss, And Long-Term Health* (Dallas: BenBella Books, 2006): 74.

[91] John McDougall and Mary McDougall, *The Healthiest Diet on the Planet: Why the Foods You Love—Pizza, Pancakes, Potatoes, Pasta, and More—Are the Solution to Preventing Disease and Looking and Feeling Your Best* (San Francisco: HarperOne, 2016): 20.

[92] Joel Fuhrman, *Eat to Live: The Amazing Nutrient-Rich Program for Fast and Sustained Weight Loss* (Little, Brown Spark, 2011): 81-111.

additional assaults that can lead to cognitive disability.

Are you wondering why you should avoid salt after your head injury? Devi Mohan, Kwong Hsia Yap et al. stated in their article, "Link Between Dietary Sodium Intake, Cognitive Function and Dementia Risk in Middle-Aged and Older Adults: Systematic Review," that "high sodium intake is associated with hypertension and cardiovascular disease (both are linked to dementia), generating numerous recommendations for salt reduction to improve cardiovascular health."[93] They further explain that findings suggest a link between diets high in salt and poor cognitive function.

While I was recovering from my head injury, I mostly avoided salt because it limited my taste buds from enjoying the full flavor of my vegetables and fruit. Plus, eating processed foods make me crave even more processed foods. Staying away from salt and processed foods makes it easier for me to continue choosing more nutrient-dense foods of a plant-based diet.

Even healthy people avoid sugar, but after a head injury it becomes more important. In their article, "Total Sugar Intake and Cognition in Community-Dwelling Older Adults," Christopher N. Ford and colleagues concluded, "There is some evidence to suggest that sugar intake may adversely affect cognitive function over time, and it may increase risk of Alzheimer's dementia."[94]

---

[93] Devi Mohan et al., "Link Between Dietary Sodium Intake, Cognitive Function and Dementia Risk in Middle-Aged and Older Adults: Systematic Review," *Journal of Alzheimer's Disease* 76, no. 4 (2020): 1347.

[94] Christopher N. Ford et al., "Total Sugar Intake and Cognition in Community-Dwelling Older Adults," *Alzheimer's and Dementia* 17, no. S10 (December 2021): 1, https://doi.org/10.1002/alz.051754.

A Picture Is Worth a Thousand Words

Me before a WFPB diet   *Me after four months on the WFPB diet*

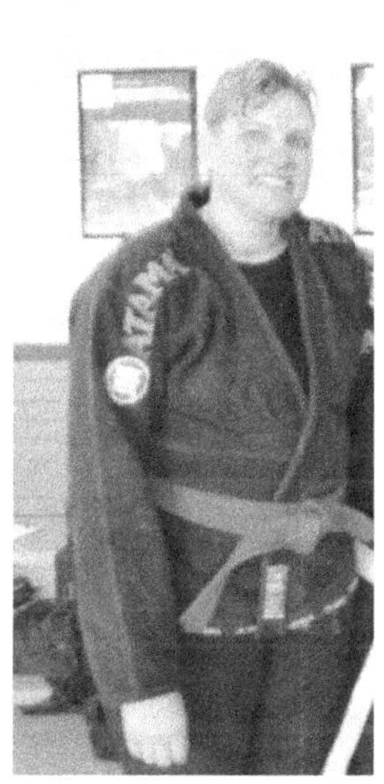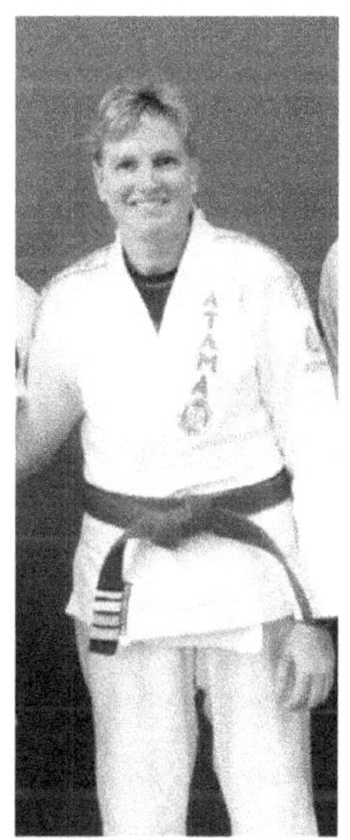

Before my head injury in 2013, I felt tired, old, and fat despite eating lean meats and vegetables and working out six-plus hours a week. I had asthma, hypertension, high cholesterol, joint pain, and horrible heartburn. I was on inhalers for asthma, blood pressure, and cholesterol medications. I lacked energy and was depending on coffee and energy drinks to get through the day. Four months after starting the WFPB diet, I lost 40 pounds, dropped my cholesterol 90 points, and stopped my blood pressure and cholesterol medication. My asthma, allergies, heartburn, and joint pain also went away. I have followed the WFPB nutrition for the past nine years and have loved the results.

Cut Out the Middleman

I recommend WFPB nutrition for all my patients. However, most of them believe the change is "too drastic." When I hear this, I think, "But isn't having heart surgery, suffering a stroke, or falling prey to dementia a drastic change? Isn't it worth it to eat more nutritious food than to risk losing your life and livelihood and becoming a burden to your family?"

Further, fad diets, like low-carb diets, don't work. Dr. John McDougall in his book *The Healthiest Diet on the Planet,* said "The carbohydrate glucose is essential for the brain."[95] He further explains that your brain operates to its highest potential when it's fueled by glucose, a sugar your body creates from complex carbohydrates.

HOW TO START

I recommend following a WFPB diet 100% of the time after a head injury. Dr. Caldwell B. Esselstyn, Jr., in his book *Prevent and Reverse Heart Disease: The Revolutionary, Scientifically Proven, Nutrition-Based Cure,*" explains that "a diet that permits even a modest amount of animal, dairy, and oil fat still feeds the habit. The craving remains."[96] Dr. Esselstyn found that after 12 weeks of following his nutrition recommendations, his patients no longer felt deprived. I, too, have seen with my patients that those who dove right into this nutrition plan see quicker results and changes and have more success in moving permanently into this new lifestyle.

My patients who opt to make small changes over time do not have the same success and often fall back into their old, unhealthy dietary habits.

First, pick a date in the next one to two weeks. This will allow you to eat the food that's already in your home, research recipes you want to try, and restock your kitchen with the whole foods you will enjoy eating.

You may need to notify your general practitioner that you're changing your nutrition if you have diabetes or hypertension. A WFPB diet can cause weight loss, which can lower your blood pressure, cholesterol levels,

---

[95] McDougall, *The Healthiest Diet*: 16-17.

[96] Caldwell B. Esselstyn, Jr., *Prevent and Reverse Heart Disease: The Revolutionary, Scientifically Proven, Nutrition- Cure* (New York: Avery, 2008): 114.

and blood sugars.[97] I recommend getting baseline numbers of your weight, blood pressure, cholesterol, and blood sugars so you can compare the numbers to before and after starting the plant-based nutrition. As you begin to live a plant-based lifestyle, you may find you no longer need some of your medications.

What to Consume

This nutritional lifestyle can be as simple as making a sandwich or as complicated as a gourmet meal. It will consist mainly of vegetables, fruits, legumes, and whole grains. Here is a list of foods you should be eating on a daily basis.

1. **The vegetables** that you eat should include green beans, peas, corn, carrots, potatoes, sweet potatoes, yams, leafy greens, brussels sprouts, cauliflower, broccoli, mushrooms, onions, peppers, winter and summer squash.

2. **The fruits** that will provide you with the most nutrition are apples, oranges, bananas, grapes, watermelon, blueberries, raspberries, tomatoes, and cucumbers.

3. If you're not able to obtain fresh fruits or vegetables, **frozen fruits and vegetables** are a great option.

4. Other **complex carbohydrates** you should eat are whole grains such as brown rice, barley, whole-grain pastas, whole-grain cereals, quinoa, whole-grain breads, and corn tortillas.

5. **Beans** are the magical fruit that are full of nutrients such as protein, fiber, magnesium, folate, iron, and potassium. Some of the beans you can enjoy are black beans, pinto beans, kidney beans, navy beans, and blackeye beans. If you don't have time to cook your own beans, then canned beans are a great alternative. Just remember to rinse the canned beans in a colander under water before eating.

---

[97] Campbell and Campbell, *The China Study.*

This rinse will wash away unwanted salt and preservatives from your beans.

6. **Supplements** are a good source of vitamins and nutrients if you're not getting enough in your diet. The supplements that I recommend to help promote a healthy brain and memory are B-12 (2.4 micrograms daily) and vegan omega-3 with DHA. I recommend B-12 because plant foods do not produce B-12. Check your B-12 levels with your general practitioner annually.

7. **Caffeine** in moderation has been shown to decrease risk of Alzheimer's dementia and to enhance cognitive function. Coffee also has antioxidants that help the brain heal by neutralizing harmful free radicals that cause damage to the brain.[98] Caffeine tolerance and its effects can be different for everyone. You will need to limit your caffeine intake if it disrupts your sleep.

8. Replace your dairy with a **nondairy milk alternative**, such as almond milk, oat milk, quinoa milk, or soy milk. You can purchase alternative "cheeses" at the grocery store, but I would recommend limiting these because they are made with oils, salt, and sugar. Some WFPB cookbooks do have oil-free cheese recipes that are delicious.

9. **Healthy fats** are better for your arteries. Replace oils and butter with small amounts of nuts and avocados. When purchasing nut butters, be sure to read the label. Avoid nut butters or salad dressings with added oil, salt, and sugar. Also, it's best to eat unroasted and salt-free nuts over their processed counterparts.

10. **Replace salt** and instead season your foods with herbs, peppers, garlic, and spices. When I need to boost the flavoring of my food, I use lemon or lime juice as a delicious alternative to salt.

11. **Can I still drink alcohol?** You should avoid alcohol early in your recovery, especially if you have a history of seizures. You should also avoid alcohol if it disrupts your sleep or worsens your head injury

---

[98] M. H. Eskelinen, M. Kivipelto. *Caffeine As A Protective Factor in Dementia and Alzheimer's Disease.* J Alzheimers Dis. 2010;20 Suppl 1:S167-74. doi: 10.3233/JAD-2010-1404. PMID: 20182054.

symptoms, such as headaches, dizziness, mood swings, or fatigue. Later when you arc stronger and well on your road to recovery, alcohol in moderation would be reasonable.

Some of My Favorite WFPB Nutrition Books

- *Power Foods for the Brain: An Effective 3-Step Plan to Protect Your Mind and Strengthen Your Memory*, by Dr. Neal D. Barnard
- *The Healthiest Diet on the Planet: Why the Foods You Love—Pizza, Pancakes, Potatoes, Pasta, and More—Are the Solution to Preventing Disease and Looking and Feeling Your Best*, by Dr. John McDougall and Mary McDougall
- *Eat to Live: The Amazing Nutrient-Rich Program for Fast and Sustained Weight Loss*, by Dr. Joel Fuhrman
- *The China Study: The Most Comprehensive Study of Nutrition Ever Conducted and the Startling Implications for Diet, Weight Loss, And Long-Term Health*, by Drs. T. Colin Campbell and Thomas M. Campbell II
- *Prevent and Reverse Heart Disease: The Revolutionary, Scientifically Proven Nutrition-Based Cure*, by Dr. Caldwell B. Esselstyn, Jr.
- *The Engine 2 Diet: The Texas Firefighter's 28-Day Save-Your-Life Plan That Lowers Cholesterol and Burns Away the Pounds*, by Rip Esselstyn

Full Circle

I strongly recommend that you start living a WFPB lifestyle. This is a great weapon to use to fight for the best recovery for your brain. It's the healthiest and most sustainable nutrition that will open your universe to a bountiful choice of delicious meals. If you need help to get started, seek out guidance from a WFPB book or cookbook. There are also numerous videos and website resources on the internet. I encourage you to give it a six-week trial and see if it makes you feel as great as I feel every day, despite having a head injury.

Chapter 23

Protecting Your Livelihood and Finances

It's sad that in some cases, missing work to recover from a head injury may create tension between you, your employer, and your co-workers. Being familiar with state and federal employee rights will help you safeguard your job, your livelihood, and your future. Your livelihood, after all, is important to your overall health.

No one is going to know what you need to continue working and studying, and no one is going to fight for you either. This means it is up to you to know and communicate your needs to meet your work and education expectations. It's also important to learn your legal rights so you can protect your employment and student status.

Get Family Medical Leave

While you're off from work, consider applying for Family Medical

Leave Act (FMLA).[99] FMLA protects your job while you're recovering from your injury. This federal law protects workers from employer retaliation for missed time at work due to a serious illness or injury.

Check with your employer's human resources department to find out how to apply for FMLA. Usually, you'll need to fill out some paperwork and submit it with a doctor's note that includes the amount of time you'll need to miss. Also, to qualify for FMLA, your employer must have 50 employees working within 75 miles of your worksite. You'll also need to have worked 1,250 hours and for 12 months prior to applying. FMLA can be taken when time off is needed, to cover your temporary, part-time hours when you're unable to return to your full-time hours, or to intermittently cover therapy and medical appointments as needed. The total time that you can use to protect your job is six weeks within a 12-month period. Every 12 months you can reapply if your recovery takes longer than a year.

It's a good idea to go to the U.S. Department of Labor website for updated and more detailed information, as laws are subject to change.[100] If your employer does not qualify for FMLA, see if the state you live in has its own family and medical leave laws. Keep in mind that when applying, some employers will let you request paid or unpaid FMLA. If you request paid leave, this usually is paid with your sick time or vacation time.

Don't forget to apply for disability to help cover your lost wages until you are back to full time. Employers may provide you with pay integration, which is when they calculate your disability benefit and use your sick time, vacation, or paid time off to cover the difference. This helps stretch out your employee benefit. Check in with your human resources department to see if this is provided by your employer.

When going back to work, it's recommended to slowly return to a regular schedule. For example, it's generally a good idea to begin with a schedule of two to four hours a day, one to two days a week for one to two

---

[99] "Family and Medical Leave Act," U.S. Department of Labor, accessed April 14, 2022, https://www.dol.gov/agencies/whd/fmla.
[100] "Family and Medical Leave Act," U.S. Department of Labor.

weeks, and then increase your time as your tolerance improves. If you're finishing the day with a two-hour nap, that's an indicator you've pushed too hard and need to back off.

I went back to work too soon, and it ended up prolonging my recovery. So while I was able to slowly figure out how to juggle my work and home life, it was a real trial by fire. Your main priority is to protect the health of your brain from any direct hits, regardless of what others want of you. Don't make the mistake of going back to work or to school too soon. If possible, don't let others decide when and how quickly you should return back to work full time. Listen to your brain and your trusted family members when making these decisions for yourself.

EMPLOYMENT AND SCHOOL ACCOMMODATIONS

Before returning to work or school, you may need to consider that you'll not be the same person you were prior to your head injury. Spend some time thinking about your work and school environment, performance expectations, and the things that trigger your head injury symptoms. These considerations will help you decide what will be necessary for your brain to maintain focus and perform at its best while at work and at school.

You may wonder when and if you should disclose your head injury disability to your employer or professors. This is a complex decision that will depend on a multitude of variables, such as your work environment, how long you've been with your current employer, and how comfortable you are with your professors, managers, and co-workers.

While attending a local head injury support group, I asked the other survivors, "Should I disclose my injury?" and I was met with a resounding "No." At the time of my head injury, I was working under toxic management, and I was aware of the distance between the letter of the law and the protections it afforded me within my workplace. So, I thought it best to keep my disability to myself for as long as possible.

The advantage of having an invisible disability is it allows you time to make the decision to disclose it or not. You should weigh the advantages or disadvantages of sharing your disability and the end goal you want to accomplish with your decision.

If you're in college, you would likely contact your school's disability services office to apply for study accommodations. In this case you'd need to work closely with the staff in the disability services office, communicate your accommodations with each of your instructors, and form a list of accommodations that you believe will support your learning. You can visit the Job Accommodation Network website for a list of reasonable accommodations you should consider.[101] Some examples of reasonable accommodations are extra time to complete assignments, use of quiet testing areas, and the ability to record lectures.

If you're employed, I recommend becoming familiar with the Americans with Disabilities Act (ADA), Title One, and your employers' policies that address medical leave, absenteeism, and job accommodations. It's the general rule under the ADA that you need to notify your employer's human resources department of your disability at the time you ask for job accommodations. In doing so, you don't have to share your medical diagnosis, but human resources may need to understand your symptoms.

Your head injury specialist will need to provide your employer with a note that supports your medical need for job accommodations. Check out the Job Accommodation Network website for a list of reasonable accommodations, and share the ones you believe will help the most with your head specialist.[102] I know searching the web for this information sounds exhausting, but you need to take control of the wheel. If you don't, you might find yourself in a situation that's going to prime you for failure.

If you belong to a union, inform your union representative that you plan to notify your employer of your disability, and include them in communications and discussions regarding missed work, work performance, or need for job accommodations that you've had with human resources or your

---

[101] JAN: Job Accommodation Network, accessed April 14, 2022, https://askjan.org.

[102] JAN: Job Accommodation Network.

manager. A union representative can help block some of the punches during your job accommodation negotiations and provide assistance if issues arise from your performance or work absences.

Consider working closely with your head injury specialist, manager, human resources department, and union representative while negotiating your job accommodations. It's also recommended to get everything that's discussed in writing. Employment lawyers recommend that when you send emails regarding your disability, work accommodations, or return to work plans, you should include your manager, their manager, a human resources representative, and your union representative. Print all of these emails and file them in your work recovery journal.

Unfortunately, there are employers, managers, and co-workers who aren't understanding when it comes to employees with disabilities. Don't hesitate to consult with an employment lawyer if you have questions regarding your employee rights. Start looking into what your legal rights are and what will be needed to help you succeed.

Legal Issues

If you're wondering if you should hire a lawyer, then you likely need a lawyer. Hire one who specializes in TBI claims. Sometimes the cost to care for your head injury is supposed to be paid by a third-party payer, such as in the case of car accidents and work injuries.

I remember wondering if I should hire a lawyer after my car crash. I'd never needed one before. In the past if I had been in a car accident, my car insurance company took care of everything. When I was told that my car insurance agents "did not have time" to get the information they needed to pay my health care bills, I was very worried after my claim was settled that I would be left with more than $10,000 in medical bills. By then I had also read three different head injury recovery books that recommended hiring a lawyer, so I did.

I used the Brain Injury Association of America to find my lawyer.[103] I called a lawyer in their directory, and he referred me to a lawyer who worked closer to my home.

This turned out to be the best decision I made in the first six months of my recovery. At the time, I was struggling with getting to work and returning home safely. I didn't have the energy to play phone tag with my car insurance agent, track emails, or fill out the paperwork piling up on our dining room table. After hiring my lawyer, they took up the fight of getting my medical bills and car accident claim settlement out of my hands.

Hiring my lawyer provided me with an unexpected bonus. I now had someone in my corner fighting to ensure I got the care I needed for my brain. My husband said at one point, "It's sad that your lawyer cares more about your recovery than your doctors." For myself, I was too exhausted to advocate for my own care and navigate a complicated health care system. My lawyer called to see how I was healing and was the one who put me in touch with the specialists who ended up having a huge impact on my recovery.

Financial Considerations

I know the last thing you want to think about when you have a head injury is money, but I'm bringing this to your attention so that you can avoid making the same mistakes I did early in my recovery.

Do you remember at the beginning of the book when I talked about your brain making bad decisions, lacking motivation, and having difficulty with planning and organizing? Yeah, so this is a bad combination of attributes for managing finances. After my head injury, I thought it was a reasonable decision to spend more than $500 on Victoria's Secret bras.

Looking back, I cannot believe some of the credit card and financial decisions I made early in my recovery. Unfortunately, after a head injury

---

[103] Brain Injury Association of America, accessed April 14, 2022, https://www.biausa.org.

it's common to spend money impulsively. I strongly recommend locking up your credit cards and having the passwords on your PayPal account changed until you're back to work full time and able to understand the limits of your financial budget.

After a head injury, it can feel overwhelming to address a pile of bills, keep them straight, and pay them on time. It's also difficult to figure out the amount of money you have coming in when dealing with state disability benefits and missed time at work. It's hard to plan your finances when there's a lot of uncertainty after a head injury regarding when you will recover and how well you will recover. You may want to ask for help in managing your bills from a trusted family or friend for the first few months or more.

Start paring down your expenses now. For me, I made the mistake of continuing to pay for things such as karate classes, which I did not attend for two years. At the time I was not aware that fatigue is a common, persistent symptom after a head injury. I also didn't think all of my energy would be spent working, leaving me too exhausted for anything else. If you have gym memberships or book, newspaper, or magazine subscriptions, you may want to save some money by canceling them until you're back to your full earning potential.

Don't plan on a settlement payment to help you any time soon either. The legal fight surrounding my car accident took five and a half years to finally settle. This left me to finance my replacement car, pay for the increase in car insurance premiums, and cover a lot of out-of-pocket expenses required to see various specialists who helped with my recovery.

Two years after my head injury, I changed careers, which helped decrease my commute a bit, but the job change decreased my annual earnings by 15%. This financial impact diminished my planned future earnings and changed my family's budget to the point I had to decrease my annual retirement contributions. I'm not sharing this to complain but to instead demonstrate how a head injury can significantly affect your finances. This can be because of a job loss or through incremental cuts into your earning power, such as missed hours from work, an inability to return to full-time work, or the added burden of out-of-pocket medical and therapy costs.

Don't Let Your Livelihood Get Away from You

If your head injury symptoms persist in holding you back from working full time, then you may need to consider paring back your expenses and planning an earlier retirement date. In this instance, consider consulting with a financial adviser.

Don't hesitate to employ the assistance of lawyers, financial advisers, family, friends, support groups, and your head injury specialist when planning your financial future. These experts and resources can also be found on the Brain Injury Association website, and they can help you make tough decisions such as possibly having to sell your home, cut back on your working hours, or make the decision to change careers.[104]

I hope this information helps you block some of the punches that may be swung at your finances while recovering from your head injury and that you find your way back to working at your full earning potential. Addressing these issues head on will not be easy, but it will be worth it in the long run, aiding you in minimizing the financial hits your finances may take and helping get you off the ropes while you fight to protect your health and future livelihood.

Recap

1. Consider applying for federal medical leave under the FMLA to protect your job while you're away from work recovering and attending medical appointments and therapies.
2. Apply for disability to help cover lost wages from missed work until you're back to your previous full-time hours.

---

[104] Brain Injury Association of America.

3. Now is the time to tighten your family's budget and cut out all nonessential expenses until you're back to your previous level of employment.

4. Return to work slowly, adding on hours and days as tolerated.

5. If you're a student, seek to apply for temporary or permanent study accommodations from your college disability services office.

6. I recommend that you become familiar with the ADA prior to seeking work accommodations.

7. The Job Accommodations Network website is a good resource for both employees and students seeking information on reasonable accommodation information.

8. Don't forget to seek support in continuing to work from your head injury specialist and a union representative if you belong to a union.

9. Hire a lawyer who specializes in head injuries when you have to navigate legal issues.

10. Seek advice from financial experts when making tough financial decisions, a career change, and plans for your future and retirement.

Section V

Getting Back to Life

Chapter 24

Getting Back Behind the Wheel

There's nothing like being able to get into a car, turn on your favorite music, open the windows, and feel the wind blow through your hair as the tires eat the asphalt. For me, it's always been an exhilarating sense of independence.

For most of us, we drive to get to work and school. Driving is an important part of our lives. But after a head injury, we are left without that freedom to go where we please when we please.

Prior to my car accident, I loved to drive. I even paid money to drive a race car. I remember flying around the track and passing other cars. It was awesome! After my car accident, I was keenly aware of the dangers of driving, which left me anxious whenever I entered a car. For several months, even as a passenger, I was too nervous to gaze out of car windows as objects and cars flew by.

You may also feel anxious at the prospect of having to get behind the wheel again. Don't feel rushed to return to driving. Wait until you're emotionally and physically ready and remember that a return to driving should be done cautiously.

After a head injury, the risk of having a car accident does increase. When I returned to driving, I once fell asleep behind the wheel. I also had a small fender bender when I misjudged the speed and distance of the car in front of me. That's why I recommend returning to driving only when you're ready.

While getting back behind the wheel took me some time, eventually I was able to ease back into it. You, too, will get back into the game of life, but trust me, there will be a lot of difficult things to think about. For instance, driving is a cognitively demanding, complex task that you probably took for granted before your head injury. It can be one of the biggest drains on your brain's energy, leaving you to arrive at your destination exhausted.

To be safe, your reaction time needs to be fast enough to respond to ever-changing circumstances while driving. Head injury symptoms, such as emotional bursts of anger, dizziness, and difficulty with shifting attention, should be resolved prior to driving. The last thing you want is to end up in a car accident because of inattentiveness, falling asleep behind the wheel, or succumbing to road rage. When you start driving, you'll want to save as much of your brain energy for work and school as possible. Hence, it's best to curb any additional distractions that demand unnecessary multitasking while driving. Turn off the radio, don't listen to podcasts, and put your phone away so it doesn't distract you. Also consider using a navigator app to reduce burdening your memory with things like directions.

Getting back behind the wheel of your life is going to happen one way or another. Even if you can't drive, if you don't take the proper steps and time to prepare for it, it can have serious consequences on your life.

Rest assured that if you've made it this far, you're ready to take control of the direction of your life. But your life will start making demands, and the last thing you want is to find yourself in a position where you are unable to handle the pressures of work and life while getting harassed by collections agents for an unpaid hospital bill.

Since getting back to life may be a daunting task, before I hand off the car keys to you, there are several things you may want to consider thinking about. As you dust off the grit and grime from your recovery journey, take stock of what resources you have at hand and how you will allocate them while getting back to life. As you enter the world again, below are six steps that I recommend for all my patients.

STEP 1: LET GO OF WHAT HAS BEEN LOST

On a balmy, beautiful afternoon, I went out to my deck with a hot cup of coffee in one hand and my recovery journal in the other. I started to list all the old stuff I had been able to do along with the old goals and old passions I'd held prior to my head injury.

On the other side of the paper, I listed the things I had gained from my head injury. For example, I was more creative, had more patience, and enjoyed a slower, pared-down lifestyle. Under the warm sun, I compared these lists. It was then that I realized I no longer cared about a lot of things I once thought were important.

What I did not realize at that time was that I was coming to terms with acceptance. I was accepting that I might not get back to my old self anytime soon, if ever. At that moment I was beginning to get to know the new me and learning to be okay with my new brain. It's okay to be angry, sad, and flat-out frustrated about losing parts of your old life. However, this does not mean your life is over—it's just a new beginning.

At this point you need let go of what has been lost. This is paramount and is an important first step toward recovering from your head injury. If you don't let go of your expectation to return to your past self, you will not be able to move forward. For those of you who may be struggling to let go of your old self, seek the support of friends, family, counselors, or your psychologist.

Once you have gotten over this difficult hurdle, you will be ready and open to meeting the new you.

STEP 2: REDEFINE YOUR CORE VALUES

To live a happy, balanced, and fulfilled life, all of us should be in tune with our core values, as they help drive our goals and decisions. To help you get started, here are some examples of my core values: wisdom, family, simplicity, trustworthiness, friendship, integrity, adventures, learning, perseverance, self-love, gratitude, happiness, and kindness.

Now it's your turn to make your list and see what is important in your life. What are your dreams and passions? See if there's a difference when you compare your goals from before and after your head injury. This knowledge will aid in defining your core values and get you acquainted with the new you. With this in hand, you can apply your core values to plan your future.

STEP 3: ROLLING WITH REGRESSION

Somedays you may wonder if you're ever going to get better. There will be days when you're going about your life and then, out of the blue, your old head injury symptoms return to knock your butt back onto the recovery couch. When this happens, it can be extremely frustrating and depressing, as you feel as if life was going on without you.

When these moments occur, remember that they're part of your recovery. It will not be a smooth road, so it's best to learn how to dance with your brain's recovery rather than fight it. Often you and your brain will take two steps forward and one step back during your recovery.

If you choose to fight and push your brain to heal faster, it will turn around and punch you squarely in the nose. This will also leave you exhausted, overloaded, and burned out, and it can take several days to weeks of sleep for you to recover.

I call these episodes regressions in your recovery. This is when you've pushed your brain too hard, and now it's letting you know you need to take a break. When this happens, you need to cut back on your endeavors and prioritize what you need to get accomplished. At this point, just do the minimum it takes to get through the day. You may even need to stay home for a day or two to get enough sleep for your brain to refill its depleted energy stores.

Examples of things that can cause an episode of regression are illnesses, a poor night of sleep, emotional stress, long-distance drives, travel, prolonged computer work, long study sessions, large social gatherings, surgery, and medical procedures. To minimize the severity of a regressive episode, plan extra sleep and rest, if possible, before and definitely after these triggering events.

Early in your recovery, it will be easy to trigger regression. As you heal, your triggers may change from simply doing more than one complex task a day to traveling out of the state for a business seminar. Once you learn what your current biggest brain-draining activities are, the better you can plan for them and the energy they will require.

For instance, maybe before your head injury a visit to your dentist was no problem for you. However, since your head injury, you may find you need a two-hour nap to recover after seeing your dentist. Knowing this will allow you to schedule your appointment according to your brain's needs, such as requesting to be scheduled for the last appointment of the day and going home to rest instead of returning to work or school.

I've learned the hard way that my brain needs extra time to recover from previously benign activities. If I do not pad my plans with extra time to rest and recoup, I will find myself regressing and needing several days of extra rest and sleep to get my brain functioning at its previous level.

It's a bummer when regression occurs during your recovery, but remember it is a normal part of the healing process. Over time you'll learn to sense an approaching episode and what triggers your regression. The keys are to be flexible with your recovery, to be kind to yourself and your brain when regression happens, and to take it easy and pamper yourself whenever it's needed. In time you'll find the balance between pushing yourself and your brain to grow, but not so hard that you're sidelined for weeks.

STEP 4: CREATE A SUPPORTIVE TEAM

While you're recovering from a head injury, you'll want to avoid any unnecessary stress or drama in your life. As you know, stress is a huge brain drain. At this time you need to be selfish. Yes, I'm giving you permission to be selfish! Your main priority will be protecting your brain's health and function so you can continue to work, study, and live life to the fullest. That means you need to be surrounded by family and friends who understand and are willing to support the new you.

Working and studying while your brain heals may leave you with little energy for friends, family, and spending time with your kids. After a head injury, it can also be difficult to find the energy and motivation to help with household chores, childcare, and family finances—let alone keeping a social life.

After a head injury, you'll discover who your real friends are. These supportive and understanding people will become your most treasured companions. Realize, too, that you may lose some friends after a head injury. Some friends will not understand why you don't want to go out for drinks after work or eat at a loud restaurant, or why you decline to see action movies in the theater. Some people may not be able to adjust to your new personality or outlook on life. Don't bother with people who tell you that you look fine, deny the significance of your injury, or are impatient with your recovery. Don't lament over these fair-weather friends. They're not worth the energy.

It's okay to make your recovery your number-one priority and to distance yourself from or even let go of family members who are only bringing stress and drama into your life. Saying no to others, slowing down your pace, and paring down your life to protect your brain is okay.

"For better or for worse" is what my husband and I promised each other the day we were married. The next several years after my head injury were some of the worst times we've had to endure. This may be the case for you. If so, good communication between you and your partner will be paramount to ensure you both make it through this devastating event in your lives. I've found it helpful to warn my husband if I'm having a bad brain day. This way he knows not to take my grumpiness personally or to rely on me to help a lot around the house.

Parenting roles or your role in the family may change because of your head injury. I found that being honest and explaining to my kids what happened to me and how my brain works differently helped everyone to cope with these changes. To this day I continue to keep an open dialogue with my kids on how I am doing or if I'm struggling with a bad brain day.

If your family is struggling with these changes, consider seeking family counseling or attending support groups. You may be able to find a support group for you, your partner, and your children, if needed. I found a local support group from the website of the Brain Injury Association of America.

STEP 5: PROTECT YOUR COGNITIVE FUNCTION

After a head injury, it's imperative to protect your cognitive function so that you can enjoy a long, healthy, and active life. Previously in this book I discussed that you have a higher risk of developing neurodegenerative disease such as Alzheimer's dementia following a head injury.

Here are five tips to help prevent dementia:[105]

- Get seven to nine hours of sleep every night.
- Eat a WFPB diet.
- Exercise and be active, either with gardening or going on a walk outside.
- Be social by maintaining connections with family, friends, and people in your community. This can be done as easily as calling a

---

[105] "Can Dementia Be Prevented?," NHS, modified June 26, 2020, https://www.nhs.uk/conditions/dementia/dementia-prevention/.

friend on the phone, sending a letter or email, or volunteering for your favorite local organizations.

- Continue learning new things. Learning something new can simply be trying a new recipe. You can also consider more challenging things, such as learning a new language, musical instrument, hobby, craft, or traveling to another country.

STEP 6: HAVE HOPE

If you made it to the end of this book, you should pat yourself on the back. You have demonstrated to yourself that you're determined to not let your head injury knock you down and keep you from standing up again. Recovering from a head injury is hard, and it may take you years to recover. It takes a strong sense of perseverance, flexibility, and a desire to heal. You should be proud of your inner strength and the work you have done to support your brain's healing.

My head injury was the start of a new life and personal journey of self-rediscovery. Was this easy for me? Hell no! My recovery sucked. It has been a longer journey than I thought it would be. Even now I get bummed out when I don't have enough energy to do all the things I want to do, and it's a journey I am still traveling.

I've learned from my head injury that time equates to healing and that accepting change should be embraced. As time passed, I developed a calm perspective for how to live and thrive within my limits. With that, I developed kindness and patience for myself and others.

I wrote this book in hopes that it will help pave a smoother road to recovery for you. I shared my story so you can avoid making the mistakes I did. I also wanted to share with you that yes, there's hope, and in time your brain will get better.

Your recovery will be as unique as your personality. Your journey may be short or over several years. Now you have tools, strategies, a list of specialists to seek, a healthy brain lifestyle to embrace, and the knowledge required to take the necessary steps to get back into life. I hope the things I've shared with you in this book will help you continue to work, study, and live to your fullest potential. Now I'm passing the baton off to you. It's your turn to discover the new you, to learn to love your new brain, and to walk your own path to recovery.

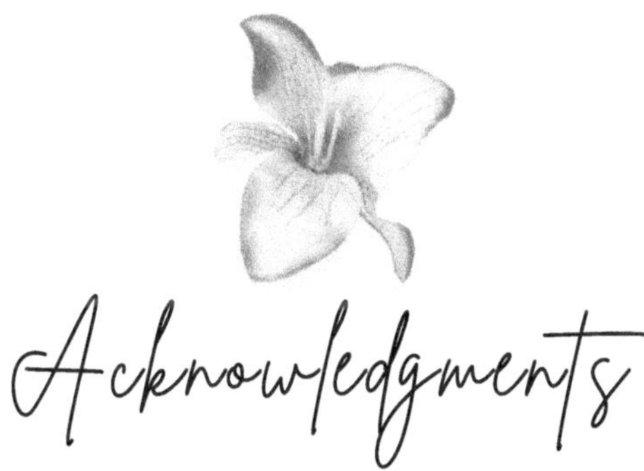

Acknowledgments

This book was written with the loving support and encouragement of my best friend and husband, Edward. Thanks to my children, Aria and Salem for patiently providing me uninterrupted time to write this book. I also want to thank my husband and children for finding the strength to carry on without me while I was broken, sidelined, and trying to heal. I will never forget how you were there for me.

I want to thank my parents, Jim and Joyce, for comforting me with reassuring words that I would get better and write this book. Thanks to my sister, Karen who calmly reminded me endlessly, "hey, you can do this". Big thanks to my friends Lesa and Ann, who emphatically insisted I should write this book and share my story. Thanks to my friend, Joanne, who inspired me to be relentless in my recovery and tell the truth with grace.

AFTER *the* CRASH:

HOW TO KEEP YOUR JOB, STAY IN SCHOOL, AND LIVE LIFE AFTER A BRAIN INJURY

 To learn more coping steps to keep your job, stay in school, and live life after a brain injury, check out: **kellytuttle.org**

 For **special discounts** or bulk purchases, contact us at **kellytuttle.org**

 Let's continue the journey! Join us at **kellytuttle.org**

CONNECT WITH OUR COMMUNITY

@brain_np_

/Kelly Tuttle

@BrainLovingNP

/Kelly Tuttle

THANK YOU FOR READING!

If **After the Crash** was helpful, please leave a review on Goodreads or on the retailer site where you purchased this book and help me reach more readers like you!

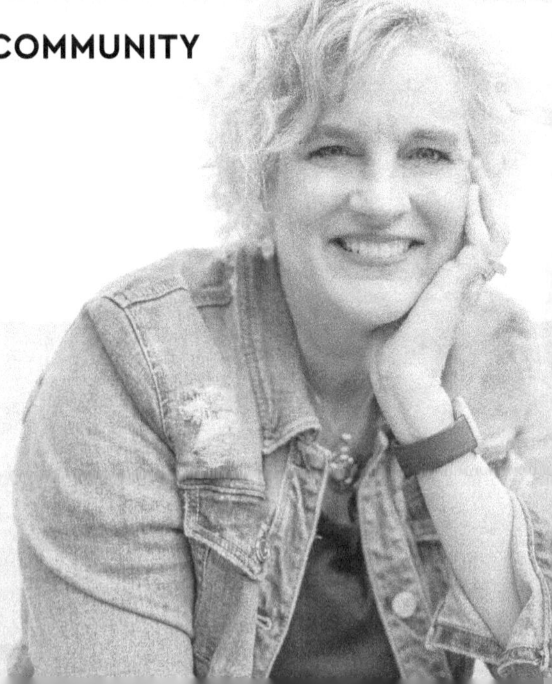